The Clinician's Guide to
Surviving IT

Alan Gillies

Professor of Information Management
Lancashire School of Health and Postgraduate Medicine
University of Central Lancashire

Foreword by
Glyn Hayes

Radcliffe Publishing
Oxford • Seattle

Radcliffe Publishing Ltd
18 Marcham Road
Abingdon
Oxon OX14 1AA
United Kingdom

www.radcliffe-oxford.com
Electronic catalogue and worldwide online ordering facility.

British Library Cataloguing in Publication Data

A catalogue record for this book is available from the British Library.

ISBN-10 1 85775 797 1
ISBN-13 978 1 85775 797 2

Typeset by Anne Joshua & Associates, Oxford
Printed and bound by TJ International Ltd, Padstow, Cornwall

Contents

Foreword

The Government thinks IT is good for healthcare. Managers think IT is good for healthcare. The technologists think IT is good for healthcare. The problem is that many of those who deliver healthcare, the clinicians, have yet to be convinced. Clinicians are only really concerned with delivering good quality individual patient care. They have been doing so for many years without the need for IT so why should they give up their time and energy in finding out about IT? After all it is mainly for administrative purposes and can even be used to observe and control them.

This book is to dispel both the myth that IT does not affect individual patient care and to overcome the natural worries of clinicians about its use and their need to change to adopt this new revolution. And a revolution is what it is. Many, many billions of pounds are being spent on IT by all governments worldwide. They would not do this if there was not good evidence that IT can improve things. Such large investment has to mean change. Different ways of working, different problems and solutions and different things to learn. Those who do understand this revolution believe it will be as significant to healthcare delivery as the invention of the stethoscope or the discovery of antibiotics.

The author does not assume any prior knowledge of IT or interest in IT. This is a book for those who realise there is something here that they need to understand and that will affect their work in the future. It is designed to illuminate the problems and possibilities for the practising clinician. Although there is discussion of the relevant technical issues, it is written to put everything into a clinical context. The examples are simple but relevant and there is a wealth of reference material for those who wish to explore further. Indeed, readers are encouraged to use the web to find out more. For those who are as yet uncertain about the Internet, there are simple explanations to get you started.

It is of relevance to all clinicians. Although many of the examples are from primary care this is just because primary care in England has more experience than other parts of the health service. Nurses, professions allied to medicine and doctors will benefit from this text. Also, although the English National Programme for IT is used to explain much, it is equally relevant to other countries that have different strategies for introducing IT. The lessons are the same the world over.

The author is a well-respected figure in the world of health informatics. The academic unit he runs is at the forefront of education and training of clinical staff. He has used this long experience to create a book which is simple to use and yet can bring the reader right up to date about the way healthcare is changing. If you realise that this revolution is one you have to get to grips with, but are unsure how to do so, then this book is for you.

Glyn Hayes
Family Physician
Chair, Health Informatics Forum of the British Computer Society
President, UK Council for Health Informatics Professions
President Primary Health Care Specialist Group of the BCS
January 2006

Preface

About this book

This book is designed for clinicians, especially those who are nervous or just plain angry about the information technology that is being introduced into the NHS. It starts by explaining what IT can do for clinicians and patients. However, it recognises that there is no such thing as a free lunch, and goes on to outline clinician responsibilities towards the technology, what is needed to keep patients safe and to provide the best possible care for patients.

Throughout the book you will encounter a mime artist who is designed to supply you with tips, warnings, things to think about and things to make you smile:

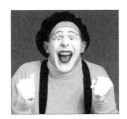

Smile!

These are designed to make you smile.

Of course, they may not work!

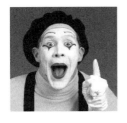

Tip

The tips are small snippets of practical advice: things to do, good practice that other people have had to learn – the hard way.

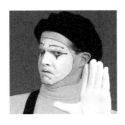

Warning!

The warnings are also small snippets of practical advice: this time, things not to do, good practice that other people have had to learn – the hard way.

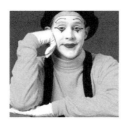

Pause for thought

If the book works then it will encourage you to reflect on your own practice. These pauses for thought will help you to do so, and often encourage you to apply what you are reading to your own practice.

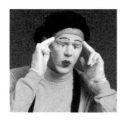

Key points from this chapter

At the end of each section, you will find the key points from the chapter. You can use this section to check that you have understood the key messages from the chapter.

By way of contrast, you will find reference in the text to 'intellectual zombies'. The concept of an intellectual zombie was invented by Professor Bob Evans of the University of British Columbia in Western Canada:

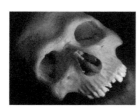

Zombie Warning!

An intellectual zombie is an idea that persists and will not die in spite of a huge weight of evidence and experience to the contrary.

The original Bob Evans zombie was the idea that private healthcare is cheaper than public health care.

To access most of the web-based resources mentioned in this book, you can go to my virtual library at: www.healthlibrary.org.uk. You may also like to visit my personal website at: www.alangillies.com.

Hopefully, you will find the book helpful – maybe even enjoyable!

Alan Gillies
professor@alangillies.com
November 2005

Part I

What can informatics do for me?

1 Informatics is important, honest

Why should we care about informatics?

There are people who believe that we should care about IT because it is IT, and therefore it is wonderful. They generally wear anoraks, collect locomotive numbers and talk fluent Hungarian. For the rest of us, we care about things that make our lives better, easier or occasionally – just more fun.

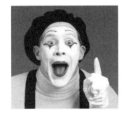

Tip: Informatics and IT

IT stands for information technology. In this book we shall use the term 'informatics' a lot instead. Health informatics, the application of IT within healthcare, has been defined as:

'The knowledge, skills and tools which enable information to be collected, managed, used and shared to support the delivery of healthcare and to promote health'.

In other words, it's not just about computers!

For many people, their experience with trying to use information within the health sector has been one of frustration, and can be summed up in the following (bad) joke:

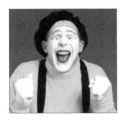

Smile!

I say, I say, I say, why do clinical staff think health information systems are like elephants?

I don't know. Why do clinical staff think health information systems are like elephants?

Because you feed lots of stuff in, most of it gets lost in its gizzards, and generally what comes out is a pile of dung . . .

However, it doesn't have to be like this. Informatics has the potential to help us do many desirable things:

- provide accurate information at the point where it is needed
- remove the need to keep recording the same data again and again and again
- facilitate joined-up care
- help clinicians and patients make better decisions
- eliminate transcription errors
- improve decision making
- manage a patient journey to reduce delays.

In the past, enthusiasts have tended to create the impression that these things will happen without effort, and the benefits of the technology have been rather oversold. On the other hand, information technology is in widespread use already in the NHS.

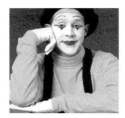

Pause for thought

What percentage of prescriptions in primary care are issued with the help of computer systems and the protection that is offered through decision support?

- < 25%
- 25–50%
- 51–89%
- > 90%

The answer to this question is > 90%. It is a routine part of primary care.
    In reality, IT brings no benefit by itself.

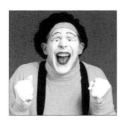

Smile!

You knew that, didn't you?

This could be a very short book, but please let me finish this point.

The benefits accrue from working in different ways facilitated by the technology. This means that you will have to change the ways in which you work. That's the bad news. The good news is that through that change, you will get to a better place.

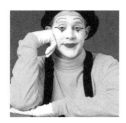

Pause for thought

'*An educated workforce is liberated by new technology; an ill-educated workforce is enslaved by it*'.

It's your choice!

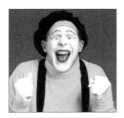

Smile!

Or if that's a bit heavy, remember Winnie-the-Pooh:

'*Here is Edward Bear, coming downstairs now, bump, bump, bump, on the back of his head, behind Christopher Robin.*
    It is, as far as he knows, the only way of coming downstairs, but sometimes he feels that there really is another way, if only he could stop bumping for a moment and think of it'.

Winnie-the-Pooh, AA Milne

Why do our leaders care about informatics?

Our leaders may have a rather different agenda. All first-world national healthcare systems face a range of challenges:

- ageing population which may increase healthcare needs
- reduced working population generating income to pay for health and care systems
- increasingly sophisticated health technology, which is generally more expensive
- people living longer, so consuming healthcare resources for longer.

Traditionally, healthcare expenditure is calculated as the percentage of the national wealth, measured as gross national product (GNP). Considered in this way, healthcare costs are rising all over the world.

    Faced with such challenges, governments are seeking ways to ensure that their healthcare system remains economically viable. In the UK, the Treasury commissioned a report from Derek Wanless, an economist, on the future sustainability of the NHS.

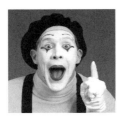

Tip: Finding information

Like many government reports and documents, the Wanless reports (there are two!) are available on the World Wide Web.

If you don't know how to find them, try my virtual library at www.healthlibrary.org.uk and look for the NHS policy documents section.

Mr Wanless reported that the NHS would be viable, provided that it worked smarter (although it took him a lot of words to reach this conclusion!).

> The Review's projections incorporate a doubling of spending on ICT to fund ambitious targets of the kind set out in the NHS Information Strategy. To avoid duplication of effort and resources and to ensure that the benefits of ICT integration across health and social services are achieved, the Review recommends that stringent standards should be set from the centre to ensure that systems across the UK are fully compatible with each other.
>
> The Review recommends that a more effective partnership between health professionals and the public should be facilitated, for example, by:
>
> • development of improved health information to help people engage with their care in an informed way.
>
> *Source*: Wanless, 2002

So, the government sees IT as a way of enabling the NHS to work smarter by:

• reducing waste
• reducing duplication of effort
• reducing staff
• replacing expensive roles with cheaper roles plus decision support
• reducing adverse events.

Frankly, you may or may not believe that this is true. What it means for clinicians is that the government is pouring money into IT in the NHS. This creates opportunities for you to use it for improving your own situation, irrespective of anyone else's agenda.

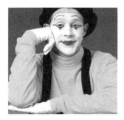

Pause for thought

One of the really positive aspects of the use of IT in the NHS is the potential to achieve health and economic goals at the same time. For example:

- increasing immunisation rates
- reducing prescribing errors
- managing conditions in primary care and preventing secondary admissions

can all be facilitated by proper use of IT and provide better care and save money.

Does it really work?

So it can work, but does it work? We are still in reality in the early stages of making good use of IT in the health sector, but already there are examples where better information has facilitated an improvement in healthcare. In many but not all cases, this has been facilitated by the use of technology to provide that information.

Case study I   Health promotion

In the 1990 GP Contract, a new emphasis was placed upon health promotion. This was facilitated by incentive payments to GP practices that met targets for screening and immunisation activity. Early examples were cervical screening and child immunisations. This was often accompanied by subsidies to practices to purchase computer systems.

Peto (2004) argued that the cervical screening programme established in 1988 has prevented an epidemic of cervical cancer cases:

Cervical cancer mortality in England and Wales in women younger than 35 years rose three-fold from 1967 to 1987. By 1988, incidence in this age-range was among the highest in the world despite substantial opportunistic screening. Since national screening was started in 1988, this rising trend has been reversed.

Cervical screening has prevented an epidemic that would have killed about one in 65 of all British women born since 1950 and culminated in about 6000 deaths per year in this country. However, these estimates are subject to substantial uncertainty, particularly in relation to the effects of oral contraceptives and changes in sexual behaviour. Eighty per cent or more of these deaths (up to 5000 deaths per year) are likely to be prevented by screening, which means that about 100 000 (one in

80) of the 8 million British women born between 1951 and 1970 will be saved from premature death by the cervical screening programme at a cost per life saved of about £36 000. The birth cohort trends also provide strong evidence that the death rate throughout life is substantially lower in women who were first screened when they were younger.

Source: The Lancet 2004; **364**: 249–56

Although some small practices ran very effective screening programmes without computers, such a large-scale screening programme would not have been feasible without the widespread growth of computers in primary care.

Case study 2   Computerised guidelines

Computerised guidelines offer benefits to help the NHS deliver consistent high-quality treatment. For example:

Stockport Primary Care Trust is tackling heart disease in an aggressive and co-ordinated way. All of the PCT's 59 practices have developed validated CHD registers, and are now implementing guidelines for managing CHD and hypertension. This activity has been supported by dedicated CHD facilitators, the production of a detailed handbook covering disease register development and treatment guidelines, and the use of computerised templates for decision support and data recording. Central to the success of the programme have been financial incentives, combined with intensive support to practices in the form of facilitation and educational initiatives, including the PCT's protected time scheme.

Source: Modernisation Agency website

Through implementation of the National Service Framework, the Department of Health calculates a reduction in mortality from coronary heart disease of 27% from 1996 to 2004. Many of the risk factors are managed through computerised screening such as that described above.

Case study 3   The power of information

In order to achieve benefits, it is worth remembering that it is information that enables change and better care and the technology is merely the delivery vehicle (although at best, it is a very effective delivery vehicle!).

A number of years ago, I found myself in a west African country in the middle of a meningitis epidemic. The epidemic started in the country next door. The disease spread rapidly in the absence of any adequate control mechanisms.

The epidemic was detected when a visitor from the country I was in returned home to his family. Unfortunately, he brought the meningitis with him and started a new centre of infection. Although he was living in a relatively isolated town, there was a rudimentary disease surveillance system in place. A local healthcare worker noticed a sudden increase in the number of meningitis cases.

He rang the central disease surveillance team in the capital, a day's travel away, and started to count how many people got ill. They didn't have any paper, so first they had to scrape around for some that was only written on one side. So they wrote on the back of envelopes, bills, anything they could find. Soon they were joined by the small team from the capital. They were able to demonstrate that they had a full-blown epidemic on their hands.

Using their very limited information resources, they were able to:

- demonstrate to donor agencies their need, resulting in an influx of vaccines and drugs
- design an immunisation strategy that stopped the spread of the disease, resulting in many fewer deaths than in the country of origin.

Case study 4   Using evidence to support staff

In a community trust in the northwest of England, the nursing teams were feeling overloaded. They had seen the number of visits rise with no corresponding rise in staffing. The team managers went to their managers in the trust and asked for more nurses to meet the growing demand.

The trust management asked for more evidence to support the need for more nurses, arguing that numbers of contacts did not directly represent an increased workload, due to the impact of other factors such as the case mix of those workloads.

The team managers were not put off and went away and constructed a workload model that measured not just the number of tasks but the type of tasks undertaken, by allocating points to each task according to the time required for that specific task.

The system was initially paper based. Using this system the nurses were able to demonstrate that their overall workload was in fact considerably higher. In response to this evidence the trust employed more nurses to reduce the workload on each nurse.

Once the value of the model was demonstrated, the teams were keen to see what else it could do for them. In order to make the system more powerful and reduce form filling, the system was computerised. This enabled the system to be used more quickly and flexibly by the team leaders. For example, it was used to allocate patients to nurses, and the system automatically calculated a measure of each nurse's workload, to ensure a fair and equitable distribution among the staff.

The next step in development was to allocate a staff grade to each task. This would ensure that all tasks were carried out by appropriate staff and that staff were not asked to undertake activities for which they were not qualified. It also helped optimise the use of available staff to ensure that expensive high-grade nurses were not being used routinely for activities that could be carried out by junior colleagues, thus undermining the case to management for more nurses.

In case study 3, no computers were used. In case study 4, initial benefits were gained without recourse to computers. Some problems, however, are complex enough to be unmanageable without the use of computers. Consider the management of asthma in primary care.

The cost of prescribing medications to treat or manage asthma in primary care is increasing rapidly. This is one of the areas that has been cited as an example of new drugs being more expensive, leading to increased healthcare expenditure.

However, at the same time as asthma prescribing costs have been rising in primary care, costs of emergency admissions to secondary care related to asthma have been falling. In order to ensure that proper funding can be provided for prescribing in primary care, we need to demonstrate that the reduction of costs in secondary care outweighs the increased costs in primary care.

This is an example of a problem that is too complex to be readily solved without the use of a computer, and without the ability to access data from electronic health records.

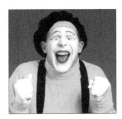

Smile!

'It is a mistake to think you can solve any major problems just with potatoes.'

Douglas Adams, 1952–2001

I'm not the kind of person who loves computers for their own sake, and I hope that we have demonstrated that the power lies in the information itself and the new ways of working that are facilitated by it.

However, there are some situations where obtaining and manipulating the information are made easier and more effective by use of a computer.

There are also other problems that are pretty complex, and cannot be feasibly solved without the use of a computer or a resident genius (and they're a bit thin on the ground).

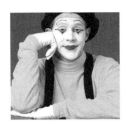

Pause for thought

Think of all the times that you use information in your job.

- Which ones do you think work just fine on paper?
- Which ones would be better if you had a computer to handle the information for you?
- What information would you like that you currently don't have, and might be provided for you by an effective information system?

You may like to see if this book changes your answers to these questions. If so, jot down your current responses so that you can refer to them later.

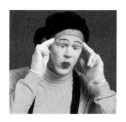

Key points from this chapter

- Better information can help deliver healthcare.
- Information technology is necessary to deliver information.
- Screening and systematic treatment can save lives; information is essential to deliver these programmes.
- If the systems are properly implemented, then they can make clinical professionals' lives easier as well as improving patient care.

2 Informatics can improve patient care

Keeping better records

Good record keeping is an essential part of healthcare and the responsibility of every clinician. Many clinicians feel comfortable with paper-based records, but there are a number of disadvantages to paper-based systems.

- *Ambiguity*: Language can be ambiguous, and handwriting can be illegible.
- *Transmission*: Paper records are difficult to transmit, and methods such as fax are very insecure.
- *Storage*: Paper records are very bulky and vulnerable to damage from wear and tear, fire, water, coffee, etc.
- *Sorting*: Paper records can only be sorted one way at a time, usually alphabetically.
- *Searching*: Looking for information can be a time-consuming business.
- *Sharing*: In integrated care, paper records lead to incomplete data sharing across multiple agencies and even within teams.

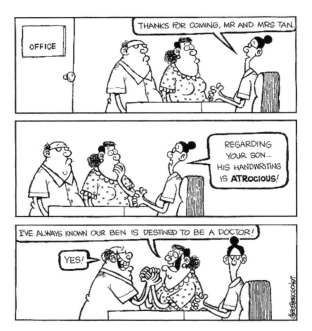

Figure 2.1 That old chestnut . . .

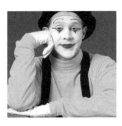

Pause for thought

The cartoon is not just there to reinforce a tired stereotype. Illegible handwriting has been identified as a major source of adverse events, and not just by doctors, either.

Mine's terrible!

The problems can be most obvious at the interface between parts of the system. Consider discharge from hospital. Discharge summaries can take a while to emerge. Recently, a local hospital told me that they had a target of typing discharge summaries within two weeks. Worse:

- they had no target for how soon the typed summary would reach the general practitioner
- they weren't actually hitting the target
- because they recognised this was inadequate, faxes were used to transmit information in a very insecure fashion.

Community-based health professionals may be further distanced as information may have to reach them via the general practice, introducing a further delay. Electronic records offer some considerable potential benefits.

- *Clarity*: Electronic records are precise and legible.
- *Transmission*: Electronic records are simple to transmit, and provide inbuilt protection methods such as encryption.
- *Storage*: Electronic records are compact and can be backed up readily to protect from damage from wear and tear, fire, water, coffee, etc.
- *Sorting*: Electronic records can be sorted any number of ways.
- *Searching*: Looking for information is facilitated by the use of structured coding schema and query languages.
- *Sharing*: In integrated care, electronic records can facilitate data sharing across multiple agencies and even within teams.

However, realising these benefits can be a complex exercise, and electronic records offer their own range of problems.

- *Ambiguity*: Sometimes the information we wish to store has a degree of inbuilt uncertainty. Electronic records can be inflexible.
- *Transmission*: The ease of transmission of electronic data can pose a threat to confidentiality and offer potential routes for attack from hackers and computer viruses.
- *Storage*: Although looking after electronic records is facilitated by the technology, many users don't do it, leaving records vulnerable.
- *Complexity*: The technology itself can provide a barrier to the information.

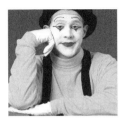

Pause for thought

What computers are good at is putting things into compartments.

Patients are complex and many of the things that we wish to record are ambiguous, uncertain or interlinked with other pieces of information.

But the same patients go down to Tesco's and shop, where the supermarket collects and stores lots of information about them, and does lots of useful things with it!

The proposed solution for the NHS is provided by the National Programme for Information Technology. You can find out more about it in Chapter 4 or at their website at www.cfh.nhs.uk/.

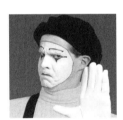

Warning!

The web is a dynamic – some would say chaotic – place. I have only included web addresses that I think are reasonably stable, but even government addresses can change.

If you come across a reference to a web-based resource and you can't find it, drop me a line at professor@alangillies.com and I'll try and point you to the right place.

Preventing harm to patients

One of the major potential benefits of using IT is the prevention of adverse events, by prompting the clinician when a potential adverse event is about to happen. Many people suffer adverse events while within the healthcare system, contravening the principle of non-maleficence: our first responsibility is not to do harm.

Computers are not psychic, however, or even intelligent, but they can prompt a clinician to act in a number of cases.

• As one example, the records hold information that show when a proposed action would be contraindicated by an existing therapy. Most commonly, this is used with medication, because this is the area where we have the most evidence. However, there is considerable potential to extend its use to a wide range of therapies.

- As another example, the records hold information showing that a proposed action would be contraindicated with this particular patient, due to an allergy or existing condition.
- In some cases, the system can highlight errors in prescriptions: for example, checking the dosage, preventing overdoses, or when a dosage is too small.

There is much interest in this area currently, not least because of the huge cost of adverse events in terms of patient well-being and healthcare system resources.

In his report *A World View*, Professor Denis Protti comments:

> In his June 2003 report, *Making Amends*, England's Chief Medical Officer reported that 10% of hospital inpatient admissions may result in some kind of adverse event and that 18% of patients reported being the victim of a medication error some time in the previous two years. A 2001 study by the National Patient Safety Agency found that of 112 adverse incidents, 35 involved information not being available.
>
> In 2004, Dr Paul Aylin, a British researcher, reported that, on average, 2.2% of all episodes (over 276 000 per year) recorded within hospital episode statistics included a code for an adverse event. His study reported that the rate of adverse events recorded in UK NHS trusts ranged from 0% to 15%. He and his colleagues noted that other studies have found overall rates of between 1% and 36%, commenting that studies using administrative data tend to have lower estimates than those based on case note reviews or purpose-designed systems. They were of the opinion that adverse events may be under-recorded within hospital episode statistics, noting that hospital-acquired infections are poorly represented within the World Health Organization's ICD-10 coding system (e.g. there is no specific code for methicillin-resistant *Staphylococcus aureus*, MRSA). Similar evidence can be found in studies from elsewhere.
>
> In Canada, according to Dr Robyn Tamblyn, drug-related adverse events are reported to be the sixth leading cause of death and contribute substantially to morbidity. Inappropriate prescribing has been identified as a preventable cause of at least 20% of drug-related adverse events. Elderly patients are at greatest risk of receiving inappropriate prescriptions. Because primary care physicians write approximately 80% of all their prescriptions for people 65 years of age and older, the Tamblyn study argued that effective interventions to optimize prescribing in primary care are a priority.
>
> In America, according to Dr Blackford Middleton, over 98 000 deaths each year are related to medical error, 40% of outpatient prescriptions are unnecessary, and patients receive only 55% of recommended care. He noted that Medicare beneficiaries see 2–14 unique providers annually and on average 6 different providers/year. Patients' multiple records do not interoperate and providers have incomplete knowledge of their patients. In one study it was shown that patient data were unavailable in 81% of cases in one clinic, with an average of 4 missing items per case. Middleton's

study estimates that 8% of medical errors are likely to be due to inadequate availability of patient information. Like in many parts of the world, 90% of the 30 billion healthcare transactions in the US every year are conducted via mail, fax, or phone.

Source: Protti, 2005, available online at www.npfit.nhs.uk

As information becomes more and more central to care, its potential for good or harm becomes ever greater. Therefore, the responsibility of individual professionals to act dependably becomes more and more vital.

How having better information available would save lives

Consider the process of providing a prescription drug for a patient.

Drug selection	Prescribing	Dispensing	Administration

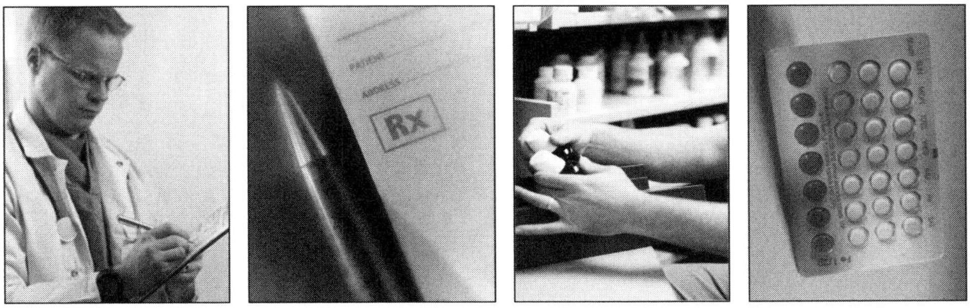

- the clinician decides that a prescription is required
- medication chosen
- dosage chosen

- the prescription is handwritten
- prescription issued to the patient

- the prescription is presented to the pharmacist
- the drug is dispensed

- the drug is taken by the patient

Figure 2.2 A prescribing process

If we consider the risks at each stage of the process:

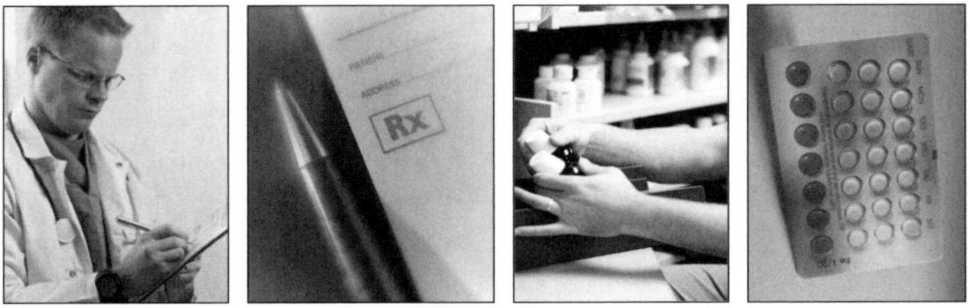

Drug selection   Prescribing   Dispensing   Administration

Risks

- inappropriate medication chosen
- patient allergic to medication
- patient taking contraindicating medication
- patient's need for medication not detected

- writing difficult to read, leading to errors in medication or dosage

- dispensing error in dosage or type

- any of the prior potential errors could lead to adverse event at this point

What IT can do to help

- decision support to prevent inappropriate medication choice
- flag up patient allergies
- flag up contra-indicating medications
- suggest need for medication

- clarity of information

- flag up potential errors in dosage or type

- prevention of errors increases chance of safe use of medication

Figure 2.3 Risks in the prescribing process

The use of IT can help reduce the risk of errors at each stage and therefore risk to the patient at the time of taking the drug.

- More information about medications available more quickly can help clinicians make better decisions about the right medication.
- Electronic records can store allergies and flag potential problems.
- Electronic records can store existing medications and flag potential problems.
- Electronic records can identify at-risk patients and suggest proactive prescribing, e.g. aspirin in relation to cardiovascular problems.
- Electronic systems can not only improve legibility, they can check dosage and other information at the point of entry to the system, preventing some types of errors.

- If the consultation venue and dispensing pharmacy are linked electronically, then the steps in the chain are reduced, reducing the chance of human error in writing or reading the prescription.
- Electronic systems can also check dosage and other information at the point of dispensing, preventing some types of errors.

Not just about preventing harm

However, IT is not just about preventing harm; it can actively improve patient care. In the above example, there are patients who will be at risk from certain conditions. Without electronic records, it is difficult to identify groups of patients who are at risk from a variety of conditions. In primary care, for example, the 2004 GMS Contract offers incentive payments to practices that manage a range of conditions. For a typical group practice with, say, 10 000 patients, it is inconceivable that the patients could be managed across up to 10 areas of clinical risk without the use of a computer system.

If the focus of looking after patients is to shift from treating illness to maintaining health by managing risk, then this must be facilitated by the use of computers to identify patients at risk.

Prof Denis Protti has reported how benefits have been realised in New Zealand:

In 1994 only 10% of GPs in New Zealand were using computers for clinical care, and GP use of the Internet was non-existent. Today, over 95% of GP offices are computerised and using one of nine Physician Office EMR systems. Almost 75% use their systems to electronically send and receive clinical messages such as laboratory results, radiology results, discharge letters, referrals, and age-sex registers.

HealthLink – the national network – is used by 75% of all healthcare sector organisations in New Zealand. Message standards have now been implemented to connect over 40 different computer systems in New Zealand, including physician practice management systems, physiotherapy systems, hospital systems, laboratory systems, and radiology systems. All hospitals, radiology clinics, private laboratories and almost 1800 general practices are involved and use it every day. Over 600 specialists, physiotherapists, other allied health workers, including maternity providers, also utilise the network. Over three million messages a month are electronically exchanged, amounting to over 95% of the total electronic communication in the primary healthcare sector.

The HealthLink network is also increasingly being used to assist with the management of chronic diseases. Common software is used to enrol and track patients on chronic disease management (CDM) programmes. The software contains best-practice guidelines for care, and collects the latest clinical data about each patient from laboratory and GP physician office systems. Based on the latest available data, the software automatically issues alerts, reminders and recommendations to the relevant healthcare providers as appropriate for and specific to each patient.

As an example, one region recognized that particular 'at-risk' groups, such as children and patients with chronic conditions were, requiring hospitalisation because early intervention had not taken place in the primary care setting. Two integrated care projects were set up to improve directly the health status of these at-risk groups – the KidsLink Child Immunisation project and the Diabetes Integrated Care project. It is noteworthy that these projects were started in a particular region that had a lower socio-economic population with poorer health status than the average New Zealand population.

As a result of introducing these applications of computer technology into a networked and inter-connected healthcare system:

- child immunisation rates have risen from 75% to 95%
- there has been an 80% reduction in wait time for statins for diabetes patients – the prescribing of statins by a New Zealand GP is typically a time-consuming and complex process; in the past, many patients were not able to receive prescriptions or had to wait nine to 12 months for eligibility confirmation; with the new electronic system, eligibility for statins can be confirmed automatically and instantly via best-practice guidelines
- there has been a reduction in the growth rate of acute admissions – this was running at 9% per annum and by 2002 had fallen to nearly 0%.

To assure the quality of the patient care process, there is a formalised, secure message transfer process. Once a message is delivered to the doctor's office, an electronic acknowledgement is generated automatically to the sending system. This is delivered either in real time or in the next dial up. If an acknowledgement is not received within a certain period of time, the sending system (e.g. a lab) will be alerted and steps taken to ensure the GP or recipient receives the result or message depending on which error message is sent back. HealthLink software utilises data encryption to ensure safety and protect patient confidentiality.

Source: Protti, 2005, available on line at www.npfit.nhs.uk*

Improvements mean change

Regrettably, improvements cannot be achieved without change. For a long time, there has been a view of IT as what is known as the 'magic bullet' solution. This myth has been promoted by an unholy alliance between IT suppliers keen to sell systems and users who do not wish to change their ways of working.

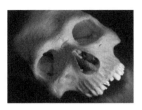

Zombie Warning!

The magic bullet solution idea (appropriately our first intellectual zombie) is that simply introducing an IT system produces benefits.

IT systems do not produce benefits; people working more effectively produce benefits.

Often this will require people to work in different ways.

An example of how methods of working need to change can be seen in the way that information is recorded in an electronic health record. Traditionally, information is stored as free text: clinicians write down the essential elements of the consultation as an aide-mémoire.

The electronic record can be used for a variety of purposes, including decision support, proactive management of chronic conditions and more, but only if the information is recorded in coded form, allowing it to be easily retrieved.

This has knock-on effects. The codes used need to be agreed with colleagues, so that all colleagues involved with that patient record the events in the same way. This can require a degree of teamworking and collaboration which is quite foreign to many clinicians.

Often, this can be a major barrier to improvements, as people are required to change the way that they work for a considerable period of time, before benefits can be seen.

Worse, if the benefit is that someone doesn't get ill, then you will never see them!

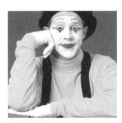

Pause for thought

In your job, think about the benefits, disadvantages and barriers associated with electronic health records.

Sort them using a table like the one over the page.

Again you may like to keep it to see if your views change as you read on.

Table 2.1 Benefits, disadvantages and barriers associated with electronic health records

Benefits	Disadvantages	Barriers
Major	Major	Major
Minor	Minor	Minor

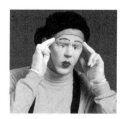

Key points from this chapter

Electronic records can provide high-quality clinical records.

Electronic records systems can reduce risk of harm to patients.

Electronic records systems can improve the care of patients, and help prevent people becoming ill in the first instance.

Benefits will only be realised if people change the way that they work.

3 Informatics can help with professional practice and development

Informatics can help you find information

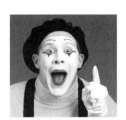

Tip

In order to get the most from this section, you could do with access to the Internet and the browser of your choice.

If this is not available, then you can still follow the chapter through the screens shown on the page.

Remember, your results won't be quite the same, because life will have moved on since I did the searches reproduced in the book.

Informatics is not just about helping patients; it can help you do your job or develop your knowledge and skills. As a clinician, you have a professional obligation to ensure that your knowledge is up to date. One of the 14 duties of doctors registered with the GMC is to 'keep your professional knowledge and skills up to date' and similar obligations are at the heart of all clinical professional codes of conduct.

There is a huge amount of information available to you, and you can use the technology to help you find what you need. Generally, you need to use one set of resources to find what is available, and another to actually access the material.

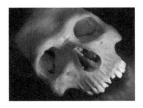

Zombie Warning!

There is a popular perception that if information is on the Internet, it is not reliable. For that matter, another popular perception is that a randomised control trial published in a major journal is Gospel truth.

In reality, these days, most traditional academic sources of evidence can be accessed online, sometimes by payment of a fee, although often the NHS has paid this on your behalf.

Resources to help you find information

On the Internet, there is a range of tools to help you find the information you need. These are often characterised in two types.

- *Internet search engines*: These are tools that search the Internet for information. Examples would be Google, Ask Jeeves, and AltaVista.
- *Bibliographic databases*: These are tools that search the academic literature for peer-reviewed articles. They are usually linked to a particular clinical community, e.g. MEDLINE is used to search the medical literature, CINAHL to search the nursing literature.

Let us suppose that you wish to find information about asthma in children. If you go to the Internet and go to www.google.co.uk and enter the search terms 'asthma children' this is roughly what you will see:

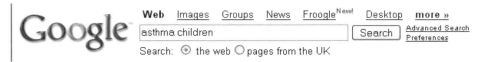

Figure 3.1 Google search terms box

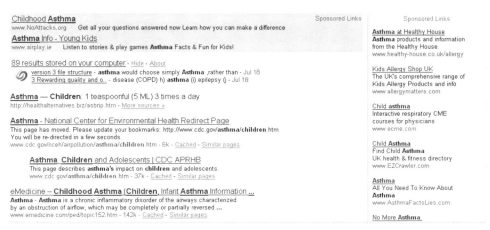

Figure 3.2 Results from Google

This window shows you two types of information. The information at the top and down the right-hand side is provided by people who have paid Google to put it there.

The left-hand column provides the actual results of the search:

Asthma — Children: 1 teaspoonful (5 ML) 3 times a day
http://healthalternatives.biz/asbrip.htm - More sources »

Asthma - National Center for Environmental Health Redirect Page
This page has moved. Please update your bookmarks: http://www.cdc.gov/**asthma/children**.htm
You will be re-directed in a few seconds.
www.cdc.gov/nceh/airpollution/**asthma/children**.htm - 6k - Cached - Similar pages

Asthma: Children and Adolescents | CDC APRHB
This page describes **asthma's** impact on **children** and adolescents.
www.cdc.gov/**asthma/children**.htm - 37k - Cached - Similar pages

eMedicine – **Childhood Asthma (Children**, Infant **Asthma** Information ...
Asthma - **Asthma** is a chronic inflammatory disorder of the airways characterized
by an obstruction of airflow, which may be completely or partially reversed ...
www.emedicine.com/ped/topic152.htm - 142k - Cached - Similar pages

Figure 3.3 Left-hand column of Google results showing actual results

One of the common complaints is that the results are very US-centric. You can fix this by telling Google only to look for the British results (select 'pages from the UK'):

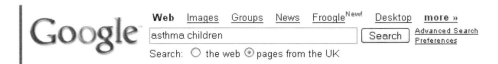

Figure 3.4 Google search terms box: select UK results

Asthma and **children**
The mucous membranes in the small branches of the airways (bronchi) swell and
the circular muscles contract ('spasm' or bronchospasm).
www.netdoctor.co.uk/diseases/facts/**asthmachildren**.htm - 56k - 14 Sep 2005 - Cached - Similar pages

Asthma (**children** under 5) - inhaler devices (No. 10)
Guidance on inhalers for **childhood asthma** - patient information, 1 June 2001. *,
Appeal Decision, 8 September 2000. *, Guidance on the use of inhaler ...
www.nice.org.uk/page.aspx?o=9807 - 28k - Cached - Similar pages

BBC News | HEALTH | **Asthma children** 'get raw deal'
Campaigners are calling on the government to tackle **asthma**, which they say is
the most common long-term **childhood** illness.
news.bbc.co.uk/1/hi/health/1965021.stm - 31k - Cached - Similar pages

> BBC NEWS | Health | **Childhood asthma** starting to fall
> The number of **children** who suffer from **asthma** and other allergies may be starting
> to fall, research suggests.
> news.bbc.co.uk/1/hi/health/2261147.stm - 36k - Cached - Similar pages

Asthma UK
The UK's independent **asthma** charity with **asthma** news, information, ... to school
can be a stressful time – not least for parents of **children** with **asthma**. ...
www.**asthma**.org.uk/ - 24k - 14 Sep 2005 - Cached - Similar pages

> **Asthma** UK - Kids' zone
> Includes news, facts and magazine articles, alongside games, ecards and a message
> board. Also includes a section for teachers.
> www.**asthma**.org.uk/kidszone/index.php - 11k - 14 Sep 2005 - Cached - Similar pages

Figure 3.5 British results from Google

This information may be extremely helpful if you are looking for information for
patients, for example, to find the nearest self-help group or to provide good
advice on managing chronic conditions. However, it is unlikely to lead you to the
most up-to-date evidence in the research literature.

This may be accessed through the bibliographic databases such as MEDLINE,
which is hosted by the National Library of Medicine in Washington DC.

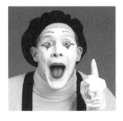

Tip

All of the databases listed below are available to you
through the National Library for Health, about
which you will find out more soon.

Common bibliographic databases that you might wish to access include the
following.

Table 3.1 Common bibliographic databases

Database	Contents
MEDLINE	Abstracts from the medical literature
CINAHL	Abstracts from the nursing literature
Psycinfo	Abstracts from the psychological literature
Embase	Index of the world's literature on human medicine and related disciplines
AMED	Abstracts from the Allied and Complementary Medicine Database
British Nursing Index	Index of the British nursing literature
DH-Data	Abstracts regarding health service and hospital administration; also medical toxicology and environmental health
Zetoc	British Library Electronic Table of Contents (ETOC) database
Images MD	50 000 high-quality images spanning all of internal medicine

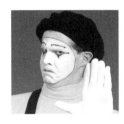

Warning!

Although these databases will provide access to a huge range of articles, they generally only list the abstracts. You will need another source for the articles themselves. Happily, the National Library of Medicine can help here too.

Type www.nlm.gov into your internet browser:

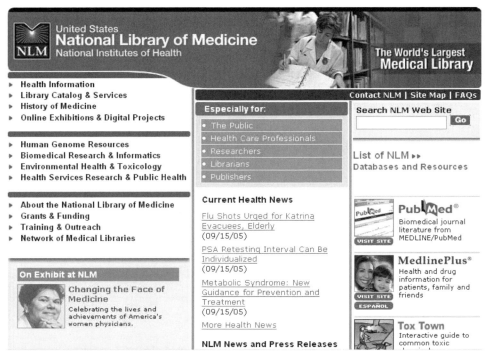

Figure 3.6 The US National Library of Medicine

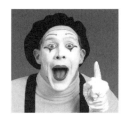

Tip

MEDLINE may be accessed through a range of portals. PubMed is probably not the best, but is available free on the Internet.

CINAHL is not available free on the web, but may be accessed through a university or health library. See below for more information.

Click on the 'Visit Site' button in the PubMed section:

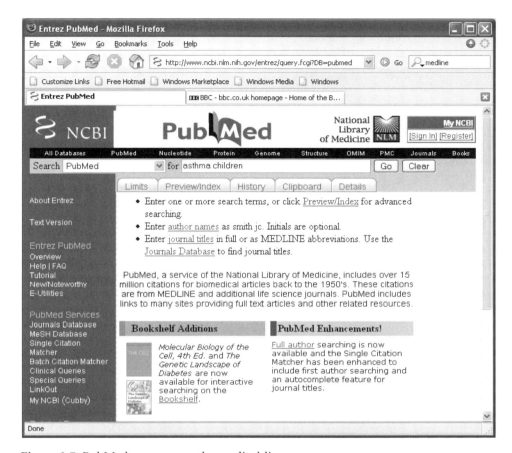

Figure 3.7 PubMed: gateway to the medical literature

Now if we enter our search terms here and click on 'Go' we get a different kind of result. MEDLINE produces a list of articles but only provides us with access to the abstracts in most cases.

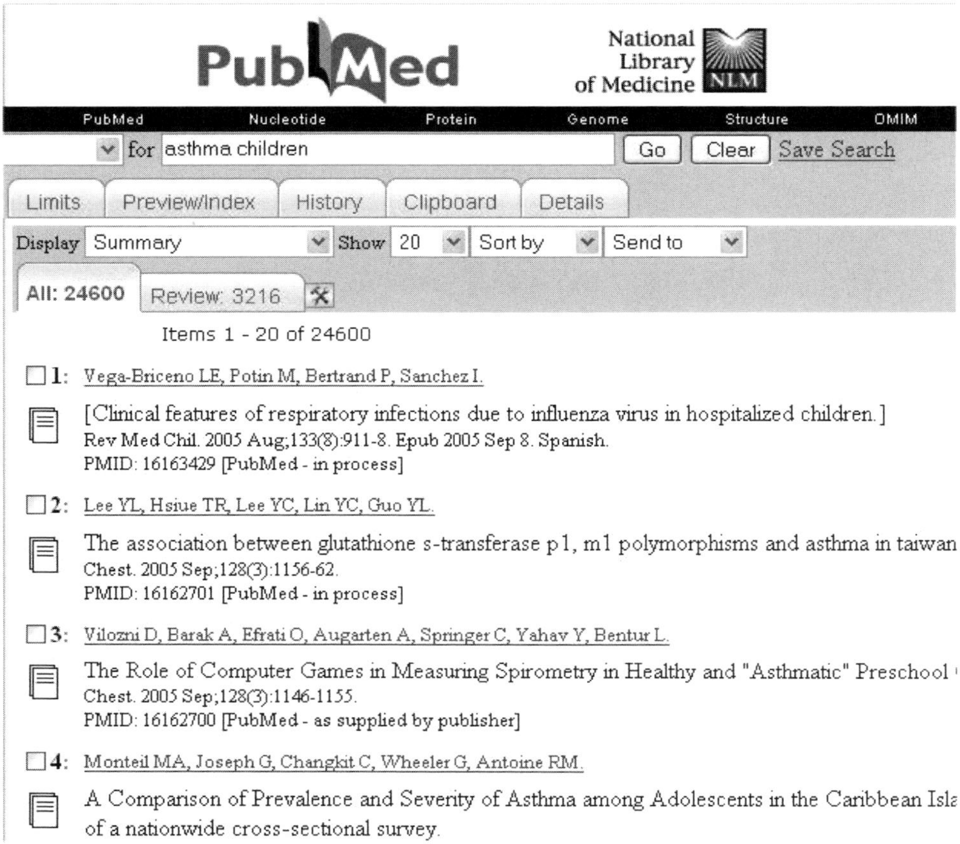

Figure 3.8 Results from Medline accessed through PubMed

MEDLINE is generally recognised as something of a gold standard. However, it has a number of limitations:

- it only lists abstracts
- it is US-centric
- it is a medical database so may well not serve the needs of other healthcare professionals, or indeed areas of medicine such as general practice.

Currently, a hybrid type of tool is emerging, which uses Internet search techniques to search the academic literature to find information. An example of this would be Google Scholar.

To illustrate how this works consider the same search terms. Type scholar.google.com/ into your Internet browser.

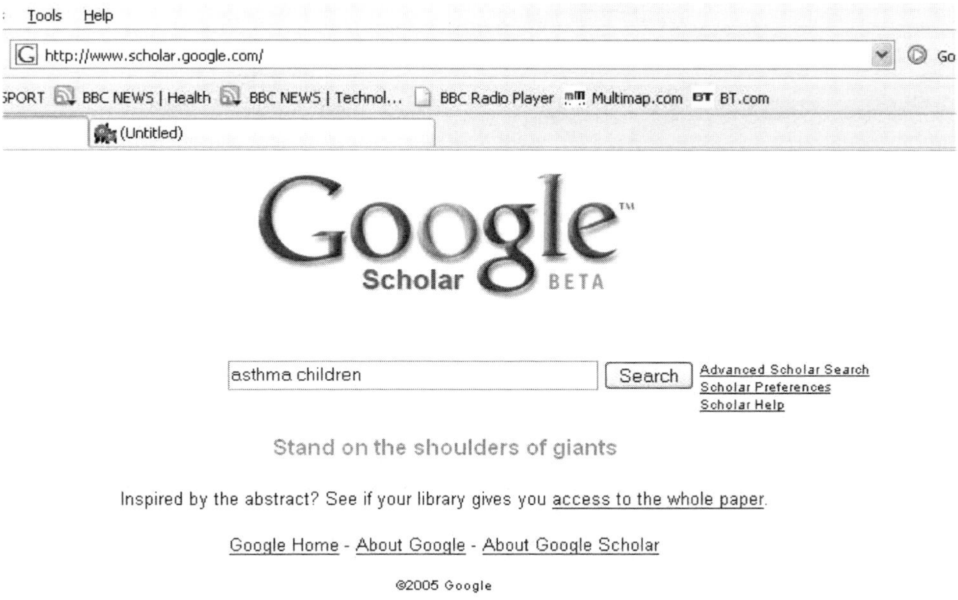

Tools   Help

G http://www.scholar.google.com/   ✓ ◎ Go

SPORT 🔖 BBC NEWS | Health 🔖 BBC NEWS | Technol... ☐ BBC Radio Player ⅏ Multimap.com ℻ BT.com

🐾 (Untitled)

Google™
Scholar ◎ BETA

asthma children   [Search]   Advanced Scholar Search
                                                      Scholar Preferences
                                                      Scholar Help

Stand on the shoulders of giants

Inspired by the abstract? See if your library gives you access to the whole paper.

Google Home - About Google - About Google Scholar

©2005 Google

Figure 3.9 Google Scholar: one of a new generation of specialised search engines

The results look like this:

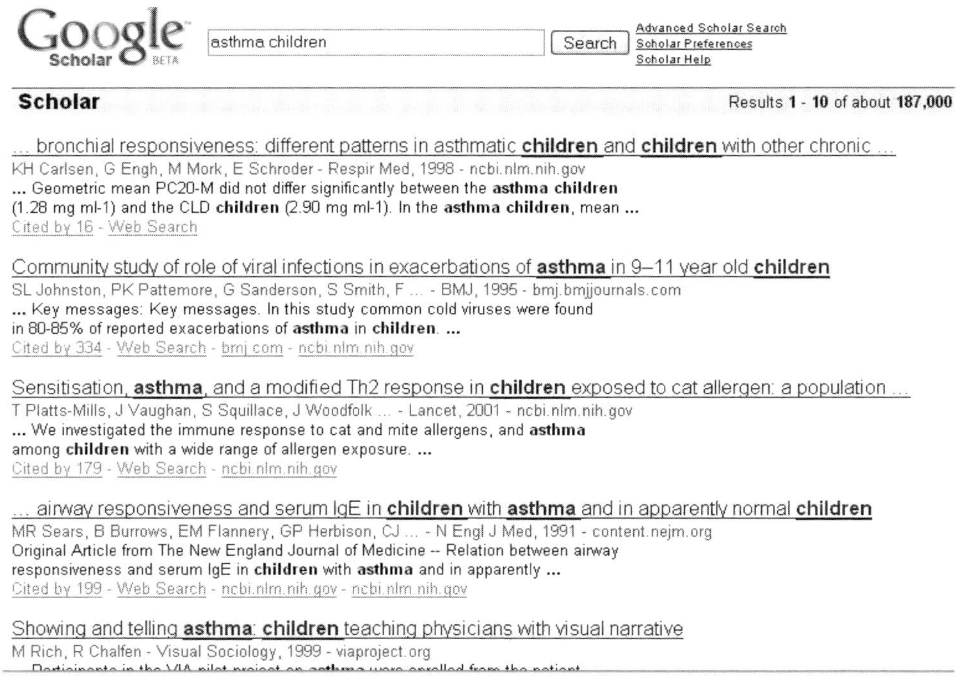

Google™
Scholar ◎ BETA

asthma children   [Search]   Advanced Scholar Search
                                             Scholar Preferences
                                             Scholar Help

Scholar   Results 1 - **10** of about **187,000**

... bronchial responsiveness: different patterns in asthmatic **children** and **children** with other chronic ...
KH Carlsen, G Engh, M Mork, E Schroder - Respir Med, 1998 - ncbi.nlm.nih.gov
... Geometric mean PC20-M did not differ significantly between the **asthma children**
(1.28 mg ml-1) and the CLD **children** (2.90 mg ml-1). In the **asthma children**, mean ...
Cited by 16 - Web Search

Community study of role of viral infections in exacerbations of **asthma** in 9–11 year old **children**
SL Johnston, PK Pattemore, G Sanderson, S Smith, F ... - BMJ, 1995 - bmj.bmjjournals.com
... Key messages: Key messages. In this study common cold viruses were found
in 80-85% of reported exacerbations of **asthma** in **children**. ...
Cited by 334 - Web Search - bmj.com - ncbi.nlm.nih.gov

Sensitisation, **asthma**, and a modified Th2 response in **children** exposed to cat allergen: a population ...
T Platts-Mills, J Vaughan, S Squillace, J Woodfolk ... - Lancet, 2001 - ncbi.nlm.nih.gov
... We investigated the immune response to cat and mite allergens, and **asthma**
among **children** with a wide range of allergen exposure. ...
Cited by 179 - Web Search - ncbi.nlm.nih.gov

... airway responsiveness and serum IgE in **children** with **asthma** and in apparently normal **children**
MR Sears, B Burrows, EM Flannery, GP Herbison, CJ ... - N Engl J Med, 1991 - content.nejm.org
Original Article from The New England Journal of Medicine -- Relation between airway
responsiveness and serum IgE in **children** with **asthma** and in apparently ...
Cited by 199 - Web Search - ncbi.nlm.nih.gov - ncbi.nlm.nih.gov

Showing and telling **asthma**: **children** teaching physicians with visual narrative
M Rich, R Chalfen - Visual Sociology, 1999 - viaproject.org
... Participants in the VIA pilot project on asthma were enrolled from the patient ...

Figure 3.10 Results from Google Scholar

Resources to allow you to read the actual evidence you have found

Once you have found the evidence that you need, then you need to be able to gain access to the information itself. This can be done through a range of online library facilities, notably the National Library for Health. Type www.nlh.nhs.uk into your browser.

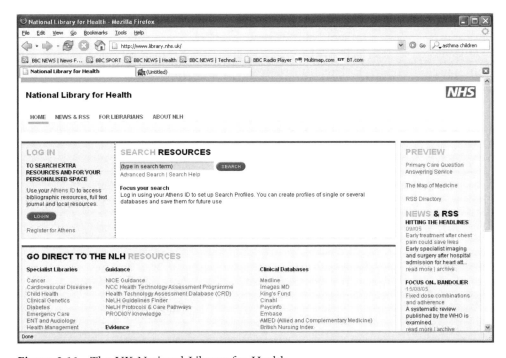

Figure 3.11 The UK National Library for Health

GO DIRECT TO THE NLH RESOURCES

Specialist Libraries	Guidance	Clinical Databases
Cancer	NICE Guidance	Medline
Cardiovascular Diseases	NCC Health Technology Assessment Programme	Images MD
Child Health	Health Technology Assessment Database (CRD)	King's Fund
Clinical Genetics	NeLH Guidelines Finder	Cinahl
Diabetes	NeLH Protocols & Care Pathways	Psycinfo
Emergency Care	PRODIGY Knowledge	Embase
ENT and Audiology		AMED (Allied and Complementary Medicine)
Health Management	**Evidence**	British Nursing Index
Learning Disabilities		DH-Data
Mental Health	Clinical Evidence	Zetoc
Musculoskeletal	Cochrane Database of Systematic Reviews	
Oral Health	CRD Database of Abstracts of Reviews of Effects	**Journals and Books**
Respiratory	NHS Economic Evaluation Database	
Screening	Drug and Therapeutics Bulletin	A-Z List of Electronic Journals
Skin Conditions	Bandolier	BioMed Central
Women's Health	Research Findings Register	Mental Health e-books

Figure 3.12 The National Library for Health homepage

The National Library for Health provides a huge library of resources available at your desk. In order to access them, you may need to enter via the NHSNet or use your Athens Password (if you don't think you have one, contact your local health librarian) to prove that you are an NHS staff member. This is because for many of the resources, the NHS has paid a subscription on your behalf.

As an example of how information technology can provide a much greater service than a paper-based solution, it's hard to think of a better one. On the other hand, the sheer quantity of information can be daunting. Your local health librarian is still an invaluable guide even in this electronic age.

One useful section is the 'Hitting the Headlines' section accessed via the top right hand of the screen. This feature provides the evidence behind current media stories about which patients may be anxious.

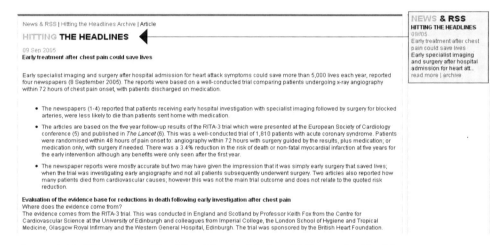

Figure 3.13 'Hitting the Headlines' in the National Library for Health

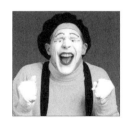

Smile!

Until recently, we had an electronic library for health, or 'Nellie' as she was known from her initials NeLH. The National Library for Health is little different, but we have lost the 'e-' bit. This perhaps represents the fact that NeLH has become accepted as part of the infrastructure, or perhaps merely that it aspires to do so (*see* p. 57 re changing names!).

Many academic resources are available online, but require a subscription. However, through the National Library for Health, the NHS has paid most of these charges for you. Therefore, in order to access these resources, you will need to register and use an Athens ID.

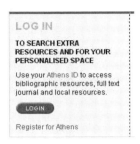

Figure 3.14 Registering for Athens: gateway to a wealth of resources

Informatics can help you present information

There are a number of situations where you may need to present information to colleagues or patients. The commonest method of presenting information is to use PowerPoint. This is a relatively simple tool to use, and many people feel comfortable with it. However, there are some simple rules that are worth following if you want to communicate effectively.

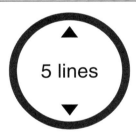

Box 3.1

Rule 1: Less is more

Never put more than five points on one slide.

If you find yourself in breach of this rule, best practice is to say less and remove some text. If not, make two slides.

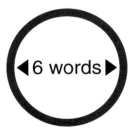

Box 3.2

Rule 2: Less is more (again)

Keep each point short: use no more than six words per point.

If you find yourself in breach of this rule, best practice is to say less and remove some text. If not, make two slides.

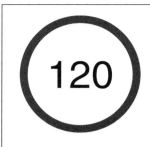

Box 3.3

Rule 3: Less is more (again)

Don't have too many slides, not more than one slide per 2 minutes talking (120 seconds).

If you find yourself in breach of this rule, best practice is to say less and remove a slide or two.

Here are three versions of a slide, all of which are based on slides I have seen at conferences.

ON THE COMPUTERISATION OF GENERAL PRACTICE IN THE UK: THE IT PERSPECTIVE
Alan Gillies MA PhD, Lancashire Business School, PRESTON, PR1 2HE

Abstract

This paper is concerned with the computerisation of the primary healthcare sector in the United Kingdom. This care is provided by family doctors, known as General Practitioners (GPs). The sector has been transformed in the years since 1986 by a series of legislative changes. These changes have had profound implications for the information requirements of GPs. They have led to the widespread adoption of computerised patient record systems by GPs rising from less than 25% before 1988, to greater than 75% by 1993.

The paper considers evidence from a variety of historical surveys and combines this with first-hand experience drawn from working to implement information technology (IT) in the NHS and through a set of interviews carried out for this study.

It seeks to evaluate the process up to the present, and to identify critical factors relevant to both practitioners and IT professionals who are increasingly involved with the National Health Service (NHS) in the UK. The paper considers evidence from a variety of historical surveys and combines this with first-hand experience drawn from working to implement information technology (IT) in the NHS and through a set of interviews carried out for this study. It seeks to evaluate the process up to the present, and to identify critical factors that are relevant Finally, it makes recommendations for both health and IT professionals on the future IT needs of general practice.

Figure 3.15 A really bad slide

ON THE COMPUTERISATION OF GENERAL PRACTICE IN
THE UK: THE IT PERSPECTIVE
Alan Gillies MA PhD, Lancashire Business School, PRESTON
PR1 2HE

Summary

- Rise in GP computerisation
- Evaluates impact of growth in computerisation through
  - ➢ Literature review
  - ➢ Live case study
- Recommendations for future policy

Figure 3.16 A rather cluttered slide

ON THE COMPUTERISATION OF GENERAL PRACTICE IN
THE UK: THE IT PERSPECTIVE

Alan Gillies MA PhD, Lancashire Business School, PRESTON
PR1 2HE

Summary

- Rise in GP computerisation
- Evaluates impact of growth in computerisation through
  - ➢ Literature review
  - ➢ Live case study
- Recommendations for future policy

Figure 3.17 Two focused slides

There are some other ways in which you can ruin a good presentation. Look at my next version of the above slide:

Summary

- Rise in GP computerisation
- Evaluates impact of growth in computerisation through
  - ➤ Literature review
  - ➤ Live case study
- *Recommendations for future policy*

Figure 3.18 A focused slide – ruined

Which brings us to rule 4!

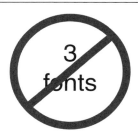

Box 3.4

Rule 4: Less is more (again)

Don't use more than two fonts, and don't mix serif and sans serif fonts.

Times New Roman is an example of a serif font; Arial is an example of a sans serif font.

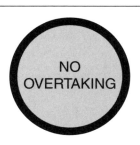

Box 3.5

Rule 5: Less is more (again)

Do not use all the same case, as it's easier to read a mixture of upper and lower case.

Look at the slides on the next page to decide which is the easiest to read.

CAPITAL INVESTMENT PLANS

- THE TRUST PLANS TO INVEST £10.6 MILLION IN CAPITAL PROJECTS DURING 2002–03
- THE TRUST IS SEEKING TO OBTAIN 50% OF THIS THROUGH PFI INITIATIVES
- SOME BOARD MEMBERS HAVE QUESTIONED THE CASE FOR PFI
- THE INCREASED USE OF PFI REMAINS A GOVERNMENT IMPERATIVE

Figure 3.19 The upper case for investment

capital investment plans

- the trust plans to invest £10.6 million in capital projects during 2002–03
- the trust is seeking to obtain 50% of this through pfi initiatives
- some board members have questioned the case for pfi
- the increased use of pfi remains a government imperative

Figure 3.20 The lower case for investment

Capital Investment Plans

- The Trust plans to invest £10.6 million in capital projects during 2002–03
- The Trust is seeking to obtain 50% of this through PFI initiatives
- Some board members have questioned the case for PFI
- The increased use of PFI remains a government imperative

Figure 3.21 The mixed case for investment

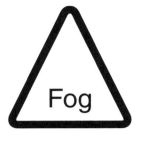

Box 3.6

Rule 6: Less is more (again)

Keep diagrams simple

Complex diagrams are illegible. They often include text that is too small in upper or lower case, and are offered with the feeble excuse, 'I know you can't read this at the back'.

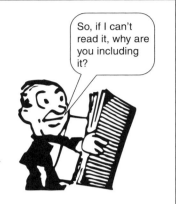

So, if I can't read it, why are you including it?

And so to colour. This is difficult because:

- I'm colour blind!
- this book is black and white.

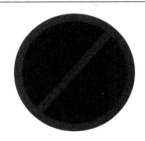

Box 3.7

Rule 7: Less is more (again)

Avoid bright colours

Subtlety is a virtue (not always encouraged by PowerPoint!). Avoid bright colours, especially in large amounts, as they can be distracting, tiring and irritating to viewers.

But it's not all about 'Don'ts!'. Here are some positive hints.

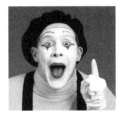

Tip

There are a number of good principles to follow.

- Ensure good contrast between text and background.
- Try near-black (e.g. navy blue) for text and pastel colours for backgrounds (e.g. pale yellow), although an available alternative is pale text on dark blue colours.

- If you have colour vision problems (I do!) check your proposed schemes with a colleague, preferably female as they are much less likely to have such problems.
- Avoid complementary colours in combination, such as red and green or blue and orange.
- Projection devices such as data projectors and LCD palettes often display colours in quite a different way from a monitor. Always try to check your presentation in the display environment to avoid unpleasant surprises!

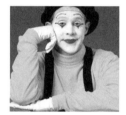

Pause for thought

If you have given a presentation recently, then how many of the rules did you break?

And how many of the good practice points did you follow?

Informatics can help you record your professional development

These days, continuing professional development (CPD) is a requirement for all staff:

> In the NHS, CPD is determined through appraisal with a personal development plan agreed between the individual professional and their manager with the commitment of the necessary time and resources. A key development in ensuring that health professionals maintain their competence is the move among the regulatory bodies to develop CPD strategies for the revalidation/re-certification of their members.
>
> Department of Health, 1999

There are a number of electronic resources developed to help you record and structure your professional development activity. Typically, these will allow you to build up an electronic record of your professional development activity as you go along, enabling you to simply press a button at revalidation time to submit your claim. The best tools will help you structure your practice and reflect upon it.

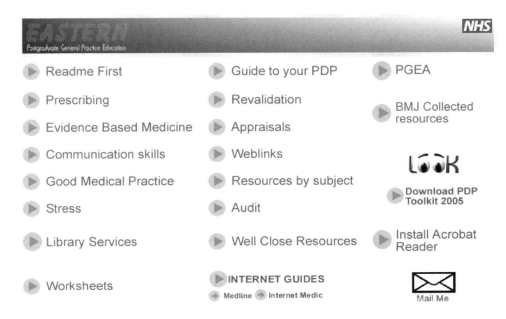

Figure 3.22 Example of an online professional development resource

You may find other useful resources under the area of appraisal, for example the NHS Appraisal Toolkit.

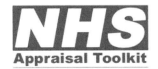

The Appraisal Toolkit is based on the principle that a single portal should be available to appraising and appraisee GPs, Consultants and Staff Grade and Associate Specialist (SAS / NCCG) doctors in the NHS in England. This on-line resource will bring together advice, guidance, best practice, practical tools and access to a community of peers in the appraisal domain. The content should be validated and kept up to date, and supported by links to 'face to face' forums and communities.

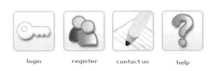

Figure 3.23 The NHS Appraisal Toolkit

So you can use the technology for both accessing information and new knowledge, **and** recording your professional development. Unfortunately, or perhaps fortunately, there's a bit in the middle you have to do yourself, which involves treating patients and thinking through the implications!

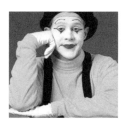

Pause for thought

What activities are you currently undertaking for your own continuing professional development?

How could you use IT to help you find relevant resources?

How could you use IT to help you record your activity and evidence?

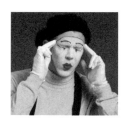

Key points from this chapter

There are a number of areas where the technology can help YOU. In this chapter we have illustrated how technology can help you:

- find information
- present information
- record your personal development.

4 Informatics can facilitate integrated care

Joined-up care needs joined-up information

One of the biggest differences between the way patients perceive the NHS and the way the organisation operates is the fragmentation of services provided. A typical patient journey through the NHS will involve the patient in interacting with a wide range of NHS organisations.

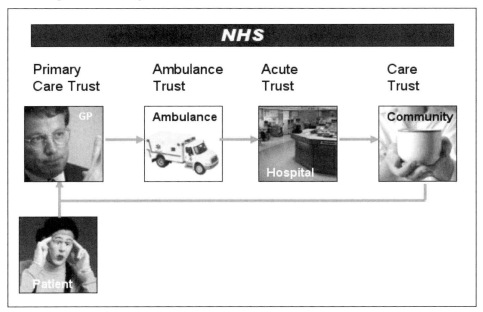

Figure 4.1 A schematic patient journey

From the patient's perspective, they have entrusted their care to the NHS. From the organisation's perspective, the patient has been cared for by the general practice, the ambulance trust, the community trust and returned to the care of the GP.

Information for Health, back in 1998, recognised that there was much to be done to provide more integrated information support:

2.31 From its inception the NHS has pursued the goal of seamless care. In most parts of the service, however, effective co-ordination of services and care has been hampered by the sheer volume of communications about individual patients coupled with the number of organisational and professional boundaries involved.

2.32 Where co-ordination and communication between different parts of the NHS (and with social services) falls down, the consequence is inevitably poorer care for the patients affected. There is also the considerable cost in staff time across the services involved in chasing up information, or resolving problems caused by incomplete information.

2.33 A primary objective of the new information strategy is to support improved coordination of care. Developing Electronic Patient Records will facilitate the shift from profession-specific and institutional (or place-related) records to integrated lifelong person-based records and provide the essential source of almost all the information necessary to deliver the strategy objectives fully. Constructing a network of locally based EPRs over the lifetime of this strategy will create a first-generation person-based record for use across the NHS – the 'Electronic Health Record' (EHR).

2.34 As a minimum, co-ordination of care must improve across the following organisational boundaries:

• within the full primary care team
• between hospitals and general practice
• between health and social care.

2.35 The inadequacies of information systems to support community health staff have been apparent for many years. The organisational independence of community NHS Trusts, combined with the reality of the extended primary care team, has in the past made the development of operational information systems most difficult. Even without the organisational changes signalled in *The New NHS*, the development of integrated primary/community care systems would have been sensible. The new NHS proposals make this change inevitable.

2.36 To achieve individual lifelong Electronic Health Records we must first develop a fully integrated 'core' electronic patient record covering both primary and community care services. In the light of the proposals in *The New NHS* to develop Primary Care Trusts (PCT), the operational information needs for community health staff will be met by the development of primary/community care systems integrated at the practice, or Primary Care Trust level.

3.6 Further development of the NHS IM&T infrastructure is required to address a number of difficulties:

• the lack of common record structures and terminology (with some notable exceptions) being used within and between primary and secondary care
• the absence of comprehensive nationally agreed standards and protocols for the capture and communication of clinical information

- professional and public concerns over the security of information in EPRs and EHRs and the transmission of identified personal records over electronic networks
- the uncoordinated approach to developing condition-specific clinical minimum data sets without ensuring there is a common core
- practical difficulties in providing mutual access to patient/client records between health and social care
- the lack of a universal coded drug dictionary
- uncertainty surrounding mandatory use of Clinical Terms Version 3 (Read Codes)
- confusion over the development of operational information systems to support community health workers.

Information for Health, Department of Health, 1998*

All the rhetoric talks of a patient-centred NHS that encourages joined-up care, but the reality too often is still care organised in silos with limited and delayed sharing of information. Consider the following case study from mental health services.

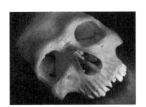

Zombie Warning!

Many decisions handed from the top of the NHS seem to be based upon the assumption that the NHS is a single homogeneous corporate body, generally resembling one big hospital.

There is so much evidence not only of the heterogeneity of the NHS, but of its significance for the success of big projects, that this is a classic 'intellectual zombie'!

A case study from mental health

This case study outlines the situation in a real local mental health NHS trust in 2001. The names have been changed, but nothing else. As with many trusts within the UK, Camberwick Green Community Healthcare Trust has just undergone a merger, in this case with its neighbours in Trumpton and Chigley; the process was completed in October 1999. The new trust name is Trumptonshire Healthcare NHS Trust. The interviews and other empirical work described in this study took place during the time of this merger. Shortly after the merger was completed, the new National Standard Framework (NSF) for Mental Health Services was published (DoH 1999).

Resource allocation for mental healthcare varies across the country. Figures published in the *British Journal of Psychiatry* (Glover 1999) show Trumptonshire, which includes Chigley and Camberwick Green, is allocated £77 per capita whereas Trumpton is funded £99 per capita for mental healthcare. This may have a bearing on the variety of services which are offered by each of the trusts. The NSF states that there are substantial variations in the spend per head of population by statutory agencies, which can be partly explained by historical patterns of expenditure, for example, the presence or absence of a large psychiatric hospital (DoH 1999). However, these variations in funding can contribute to unacceptable variations in the quality and quantity of service provided. Camberwick Green Mental Healthcare Trust is a satellite service with the old psychiatric hospitals based at Murraytown and Postgate.

The NSF sets out national standards of service organisation and delivery within mental health services in England and Wales. It acknowledged the *Information for Health* information strategy policy document (DoH 1998), but stated that information requirements for mental health were poorly provided for within the mental health setting and that mental health settings needed their own policy document regarding information strategies. The new Framework document therefore recommended that a 'think-tank' be set up to prepare this new policy for mental health requirements. It stated that all mental health services should have in place an integrated mental health electronic record by 2007. The first mental health information strategy document (DoH 2001) was made public in March 2001.

Trumptonshire Healthcare Trust therefore aimed to develop its own system for maintaining electronic records and did, in effect, have the framework for a system in place. However, this was based on acute care of physically ill patients and did not take into consideration the more complex information requirements that mental health practitioners needed to provide an integrated and coherent service to their clients.

Camberwick Green Mental Health Services Trust

The research context began as Camberwick Green's mental health services, prior to the merger. Although the study included the phase when the merger was happening, the context for the study remained those services and locations from within the old trust. The trust provided both primary and secondary mental health services. The computerised system, the CIS, was not networked throughout all services. Some practitioners worked with handwritten records, others on stand-alone PCs, whereas others were linked to the central system.

The organisation was characterised by fragmentation, reflecting the view expressed in *The New NHS* (DoH 1997), in terms of both its service provision and its information support.

Fragmentation of service provision and information support

The inpatient unit was placed within the general hospital, which was a separate trust. It had 29 acute admission beds, with no separate ward for females. There were three consultant psychiatrists. The staff complement was one ward manager, four sister/charge nurses, eight 'E' grade staff nurses, and 16 nursing assistants. Internal rotation was in operation, with four members of night staff, two of whom were trained nurses. The complement for day staff was five per shift. There was also an assistant nurse who worked 9–5 to assist with patient activities. Until recently the advocacy service 'ACE' (advocate, communication and empowerment) attended the ward on a weekly basis, to run individual surgeries for patients and group sessions. Voluntary groups needed accurate information as they represented patients regarding their care, and this provided an impetus for staff to collate information, which may be required by this service. A pre-discharge group was facilitated by the National Association of Mental Health (MIND). The inpatient unit suffered many of the general problems faced within the acute psychiatric services throughout the country and these have been highlighted in a recent publication about acute services (SNMAC 1999). The unit was open for 24 hours, seven days per week. Nursing documentation was kept on the ward and when the patient was discharged, the documentation was filed within the back of the medical records.

The CIS was networked on the ward, but the only inputting done by nursing staff was the HoNOS (Health of the Nation Outcome Scale) scoring (Wing *et al.* 1996), as the ward was taking a lead position in its piloting within the trust. The ward, as with every other site at the trust, was unable to access any other computerised system even though they used the same pathology and x-ray services, which had no interface for communication to the ward despite being in the same building.

The day hospital was based below the inpatient unit and offered placement for 10 places per day. Inpatient groups were also held within the day hospital. The day hospital ran ECT (electroconductive therapy) sessions twice per week for the whole service, which was required to report to a national data collection study at the Department of Health. The staffing was two full-time trained nurses, with a part-time trained member who ran the ECT sessions. An occupational therapist (OT) attended the day hospital on a sessional basis in order to facilitate the needs of the inpatient group who attended these sessions. The OT department provided a separate team based at a nearby hospital. The team covered both the acute and elderly services. Two nursing assistants also worked in day care, with time allocated to outpatients (OP). Both day-care services and outpatient services were networked to CIS. These services only open 9–5, Monday to Friday, with the nursing documentation always kept separate from the inpatient nursing records, causing problems if out-of-hours access was required by the services, which covered a 24-hour period. The OTs also kept their own case notes at a separate base.

The 11 community psychiatric nurses (CPNs) were based within one building, situated approximately one mile away from the acute psychiatric unit. Their main target group was patients with enduring mental illness, but they also responded to referrals from the primary care groups (PCGs) (DoH 1997). As with the inpatient unit, they worked within the confines of the Care Programme Approach (CPA) (DoH 1990a). The team provided a 9–5 service, with weekend cover, also 9–5. The CPN department kept all their documentation, within their own filing system, at their own site.

The psychology department was once again separately organised, based at a different location. The psychology services received referrals from GPs as well as referrals from the other areas within the trust. The psychology department had their own systems and did not work within the CPA (DoH 1990a), but had their own records. The psychologists offered a service that covered the hours of 9–5 Monday to Fridays; as in the case of other services within the trust, documentation was filed and kept on their own site.

To make things even more confusing, the counselling and psychotherapy teams were based within two further sites, one being in Camberwick Green itself, and the other 10 miles away. The team had one manager who covered both sites, but was based at yet another site. The counselling services took clients mainly from the primary health groups (PHGs) (DoH 1997), but also had expertise in dealing with enduring mental illness and took referrals from secondary services. The service worked within the CPA (DoH 1990a). The satellite clinic was based upstairs with its reception downstairs. Remarkably, the CIS was only networked upstairs, so appointments and referrals were entered into a stand-alone system downstairs by the receptionist. The service was offered on an appointment basis 9–5, Monday to Friday. Once again, documentation was kept separately and filed on-site.

At the time, the trust had only one self-harm liaison nurse, who was based one mile away from the acute unit. The liaison nurse had time allocated to do initial assessment on the medical wards in the general hospital and worked closely with A&E (Accident and Emergency), and the on-call psychiatrist. He did not use the CPA or the risk assessments used within other areas of the trust (DoH 1990a). He had his own assessment tool and retained his own documentation. The service he provided was 9–5, Monday to Friday, and there was no access to his documentation outside these hours as it was kept locked in his office.

The Drug and Alcohol Consortium was based on yet another site, approximately one mile away from the inpatient unit. It took referrals from primary and secondary services. Alcohol referrals were only accepted via the Alcohol Advisory Service, which was based in a different location in Camberwick Green. Patients were required to self-refer to the Alcohol Advisory Service. Once again, the Drug and Alcohol Consortium did not work within the guidelines of CPA or risk assessment (DoH 1990a). They also had their own documentation, which remained on-site. The service was offered on a 9–5 basis, Monday to Friday, with no access to documentation or services outside these hours.

The Intensive Home Support Team (IHST) was not networked to the CIS and stood as a joint team of health staff and social services staff. It was based within the social services resource centre at a different location in Camberwick Green, approximately two miles away from the inpatient unit. The team worked closely with patients, either to provide early discharge support from the inpatient unit or to give intensive support in an attempt to prevent admission. Initially, the team worked to provide weekend cover on a 9–5 basis, seven days a week, but the weekend cover was stopped, due to service changes. This team worked within the confines of the CPA (DoH 1990a) and also piloted the use of HoNOS to predict psychiatric morbidity (Wing *et al.* 1996). The service kept separate records for health staff and social staff 'for legal reasons' on advice from the trust solicitor.

The mental health social services were also based at the same site as the Intensive Home Care Team, which lent itself to some sharing of documentation and information. The service comprised the purchasing team and the provider team with both teams having different team leaders. The purchasing team completed the referrals to the service using a banding system. If the referral met the banding criteria then the referral was given to the provider team. There is no other route into the service. If the childcare social work team had a referral for social worker input, then the same referral system would be followed. The social services resource centre had close links with housing and education. They had a day-care centre that operated on a 9–5 basis, Monday to Friday. The mental health social services worked within the CPA (DoH 1990a), but were not networked to the CIS. They were networked to the Social Services Information Database (SID) and their notes were not available out of hours.

Another group of practitioners – approved social workers (ASWs) – were based at the resource centre on a rota basis, 9–5; however, the out-of-hours work was covered by the EDT (emergency duty team). Their catchment area covered the out-of-hours provision for separate services from the whole of Trumptonshire.

Police services are also involved in the care of the mentally ill. The police get involved with problems that arise in the community; the inpatient unit is a place of safety following arrest. Joint working with the police and the criminal justice system is an area of neglect, which has been highlighted in the NSF (DoH 1999). Once again, documentation did not follow the patient nor were the police or probation services linked into the CIS.

The trust had established a CIS network to facilitate communication between the dispersed locations of the trust. As discussed earlier, social services had their own SID system; however, the links provided were limited. None of the agencies outside the trust, for example, PCGs, social services, police, forensic and probation services, could access the CIS. The trust itself could not access SID and not all of their own services within the Trust could access their own CIS network. Figure 4.2 summarises the extent of integration of information support. The trust introduced the CIS to meet the needs of the 1992 IM&T (Information Management & Technology) Strategy. The CIS went live in October 1997. Prior to this, various groups were set up throughout the trust. The 'Operations Group' included clinicians from all professions and all areas of the Mental Health Directorate. This appeared to meet the vision of the IM&T (DoH NHSE 1992) to 'enable practitioners' to meet their information needs. However, it soon became apparent that the CIS was not meeting the needs of the information

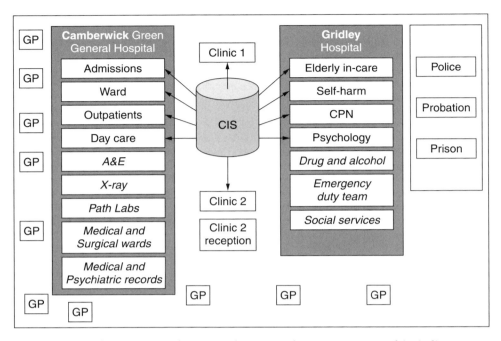

Note: Connected services are shown in plain type, those not connected in italics.

Figure 4.2 The trust CIS network as established at the time of this study

and contracting departments. All resources were diverted to meet their needs and the voice of the clinicians appeared to be lost.

The CIS, when fully implemented, did not network to all areas of the Mental Health Directorate. One of the key practitioner information needs is for timely and accurate information to support the process of risk assessment. The CPA (DoH 1990) was also introduced locally, and training sessions were provided by outside facilitators from a local university. The CPA has not been included in this new system and it is managed by use of paperwork and one stand-alone system. There have been recent improvements made in discharge planning as the trust has now established an inter-agency agreement. However, this is completed on paper with the use of faxes to communicate between each team. The use of faxes is not ideal for security, but it has become a local communication solution to avoid the delays in the postal system within the organisation.

Key parts of the system providing care to patients had no access to the system, including A&E, the Drug and Alcohol Consortium, IHST, social services, PCGs, path lab, x-ray department and general outpatient service. There appeared to be a misguided preoccupation with confidentiality and sharing information within the mental health services.

Risk assessment is an integral part of the CPA; there is no standardisation between trusts. However, even within the trust there are significant differences in the way that risk assessment is carried out. Prior to the joint inter-agency discharge planning, there was little compliance with standards of completion and adherence to the management plan. Many inquiries into homicides of mentally disordered people have highlighted the crucial role played by the breakdown in communication, leading to poor risk assessment and poor risk management (e.g. Blom Cooper *et al.* 1995). At the trust, risk assessment and planning is completed on paper, which in turn leads to access difficulties for practitioners who work 'out of hours'.

This fragmentation has implications not just for patient care, but for staff attitudes to the system. Interviews with staff revealed a range of frustrations with the system, directly attributable to the fragmented nature of the system:

- significant data duplication and multiple data entry
- lack of access to crucial information at the point of delivery of care
- a sense that clinicians were collecting information for managers and other people in non-clinical roles.

NPfIT: from jigsaw to trainset – the vision

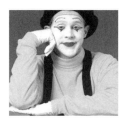

Pause for thought

Why jigsaw to trainset?

Currently we have a jigsaw, lots of useful pieces, but little idea of a whole picture.

A long time ago, when they first started building railways, Stephenson in the north built railways with rails that were 4 ft 8½ in apart. Meanwhile in the south and west, Brunel was building railways that had rails that were 7 ft apart.

If we are to succeed then we need common standards to join things up as Stephenson and Brunel discovered in the nineteenth century when the 7 ft gauge of the GWR met the 4 ft 8½ in gauge of the northern railways.

Eventually, the Great Western Railway fell into line and the standard gauge was agreed as 4 ft 8½ in.

The impetus for a joined-up national information system for the NHS comes from the first Wanless Report. This was a report commissioned by the Treasury to answer the question, 'Is a publicly funded NHS financially viable in the medium to long term?'.

The answer was 'Yes, but only if the NHS works smarter, and a major part of this was better use of information technology'.

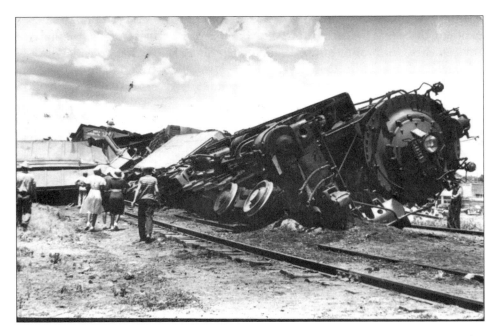

Figure 4.3 Failure to recognise the importance of standards will derail the vision of a national networked NHS

6.18 The Review believes that there is a particularly strong case for setting common standards in ICT. Chapter 3 describes the health service's very poor record on ICT investment. There appear to be two key reasons why the state of ICT in today's health service is as poor as it is:

- ICT budgets – which have traditionally been allocated locally – have frequently been used to fund other areas of spending to help relieve short-term pressures; and
- there has been inadequate setting of ICT standards from the centre, resulting in a diverse range of incompatible systems across the health service.

6.19 These points came through strongly in consultation. The Royal College of Nursing called for stronger central direction on standards and accredited solutions to prevent resources being wasted in the future, while EDS (Electronic Data Systems) argued that the bulk of NHS ICT procurement is still undertaken at local level leading to expensive 'reinvention of the wheel' and failure to take advantage of NHS purchasing power. They suggested the need to 'ring-fence appropriate funding to deliver a National Information Infrastructure for the Health Service'.

6.20 The NHS Information Strategy in England and similar strategies and plans in the Devolved Administrations have defined ambitious targets for the use of ICT across the health service. For example, the NHS Information

Strategy sets out the intention that, by the end of this year, hospitals and GPs should be routinely exchanging electronic requests for referrals, discharge summaries, and laboratory and radiology requests and results. By 2005, it is planned that there will be an electronic patient record system for all acute hospitals, integrated primary and community care records, and 24-hour emergency care access to patient records.

6.21 Chapter 3 sets out how the Review's projections incorporate a doubling of spending on ICT to fund ambitious targets of the kind set out in the NHS Information Strategy. However, before committing to such significant increases in spending, a number of important points will require careful consideration:

- the government and the health service must ensure that they have clear and well-developed views about the benefits which they want to achieve and how they will be delivered, with patients at the core of the system. The implications for staff training will also need to be considered carefully;
- to avoid duplication of effort and resources and to ensure that the benefits of ICT integration across health and social services are achieved, the Review recommends that stringent standards should be set from the centre to ensure that systems across the UK are fully compatible with each other; and
- to ensure that resources intended for ICT spending are not diverted to other uses, and are used productively, the Review recommends that budgets should be ring-fenced and achievements audited.

6.22 If these issues can be addressed, the Review believes that national, integrated ICT systems across the health service can lay the basis for the delivery of significant quality improvements and cost savings over the next 20 years. Without a major advance in the effective use of ICT (and this is a clear risk given the scale of such an undertaking), the health service will find it increasingly difficult to deliver the efficient, high quality service which the public will demand. This is a major priority which will have a crucial impact on the health service over future years.

Wanless, 2002*

The vision for the joined-up NHS information system was set out in a report called *Delivering 21st Century IT Support for the NHS* (DoH 2002).

2.2.1 Our vision for information and IT is to connect delivery of the NHS Plan with the capabilities of modern information technologies. In the sections below we set out some of the practical examples of key stakeholder experience in an NHS operating with modern IT at its heart.

The same document states that the following benefits will be delivered for patients:

- direct and visible impacts on how they interact with the healthcare system and on their experience as consumers of health services
- they will see that their health records are always readily available to staff
- they will have the chance to help maintain the quality of those records
- staff will be able to answer any questions the patients ask
- up-to-date treatment and prescribing protocols care based upon the latest medical knowledge and clinical practice
- patient-friendly care protocols will be available
- citizens will be able to obtain information over the phone or via the Internet 24 hours a day
- up-to-date information about their symptoms to be online (via Internet or DiTV)
- be able to contact a call centre to receive advice and make appointment bookings online
- telecare and monitoring services will be available from the convenience of their home.

And for healthcare professionals:

- healthcare professionals will have safe, fast, modern IT systems to support them routinely in their work
- staff will be able to review case histories, schedule care plans, prescribe drugs, commission tests and view results quickly and conveniently
- time with patients will be spent more effectively in delivering safe, high-quality care, based on universally available, secure, accurate, up-to-date electronic records
- access to research and knowledge will be freely available
- continuing personal development will be supported by a process of lifelong learning via the resources of the NHS University
- fast, secure, reliable communications links will support telemedicine services designed around patients' needs
- remote monitoring of some conditions will be commonplace.

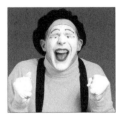

Smile !

Well you have to, don't you? Here are some of my own suggestions to add to the list:

- eliminate world poverty
- seal the hole in the ozone layer
- make everyone live happily after.

And catch that pig flying overhead!

The problem is that all of these goals are all potentially attainable, but not in the short term, not without some change and some pain. Some of the most useful things for clinicians would be much less spectacular:

- reduction in time spent entering data due to elimination of duplicate data entry and well-designed interfaces
- simple ways to send the patient's record to the next care provider in the patient's journey
- information systems that work in ways that facilitate and encourage good clinical practice.

The reality of the vision is represented by the National Programme for Information Technology.

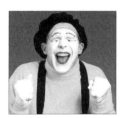

Smile !

The National Programme for Information Technology has recently changed its name to NHS Connecting for Health.

There are two problems with this.

1. Generally, when public sector programmes change their names, it's because they are either unpopular or in trouble (remember Windscale?).
2. The name is allegedly already copyrighted by an American company!

NPfIT: from jigsaw to trainset – the reality

The national system under construction is based around a national data spine to which all clinical systems will be attached. Each local system will retain its full electronic patient record, while the core of the record will be made available to any care giver within the system who has a need and a right to access the information. A schematic shows how the system will work (*see* Figure 4.4). In reality the national programme is a collection of regional programmes, each consisting of several major projects operating to common standards (*see* Figure 4.5). There are two types of providers: national providers who provide applications across the whole country, and then local service providers who provide services within a cluster. In reality, these providers are consortia of companies.

Table 4.1 shows the major components that make up the national programme.

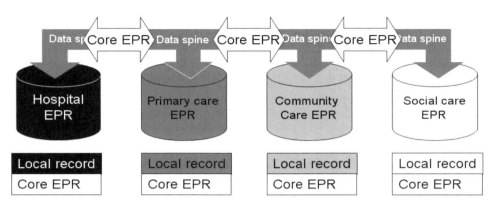

Figure 4.4 Schematic of National Programme for Information Technology

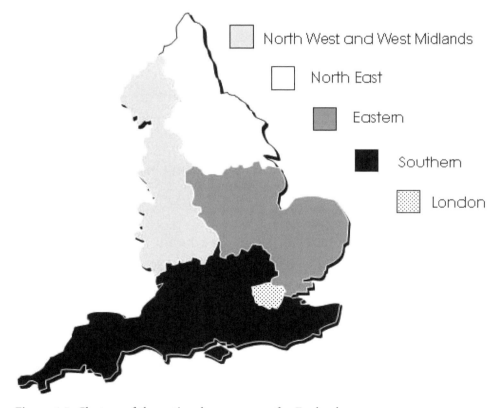

Figure 4.5 Clusters of the national programme for England

Table 4.1 The major components that make up the national programme

Component	Function	Target for delivery (as at end of 2004)
Choose and book (National)	Make it easier and faster for hospital appointments to be booked by GPs and other primary care staff at times to suit patients Offer a choice of four or five hospitals or other appropriate healthcare providers at the time of referral by 2005	Achieve 100% booked appointments for day cases by December 2005
Electronic transfer of prescriptions (National)	Transfer prescriptions from clinician to dispensary to reimbursement agency electronically in order to: • prevent errors and other adverse events • reduce administration • speed up processing	Roll-out to start in 2005 No published deadline for completion
N3 network (National)	The high-speed network to link up all facilities to provide greater transmission speed and capacity, e.g. transmission of a chest x-ray Without IT, it is delivered by taxi Over a dial-up system it takes 30 minutes Over NHSNet, it takes 4 minutes Over N3, it will take 2 minutes (Source: NPfIT)	Completion around 2007
Electronic records systems (Cluster based)	To provide electronic patient records at the point of care to facilitate: • best possible decision making • evidence-based decision support • warning of potential risks • better information for patients	Full implementation due by 2010. More detail below

Much of the work should be invisible to you, and you will only find out about it if something goes wrong. The part of the national programme that clinicians will deal with is known as the NHS Care Records Service (NHS CRS).

In addition to the actual records, the NHS CRS is seeking to deliver a range of related services, particularly a choose and book electronic booking service and an electronic transfer of prescription service.

This is being phased in over time. The promised delivery dates for the NorthWest–West Midlands cluster where I live are as shown in Table 4.2.

Table 4.2 Promised delivery dates for the Northwest–West Midlands cluster

Phase	Deliverables
1. June–Dec 04	• choose and book • basic patient information • birth and death notification • recording of allergies • beginning of summary health record • Electronic Transmission of Prescription (ETP)
2. June 05–June 06	• health record grows • orders and results for diagnostic images and pathology • support for care pathways • GPs notified of emergency and out-of-hours encounters
3. 2006–08	• support for all doctors and nurses to help with decisions • electronic prescribing • care at home helped by remote links to healthcare professionals anywhere in the community • better healthcare planning by using the facts and figures held on NHS CRS
4. 2008–2010	• final features incorporated to complete full integration between health and social care systems across England

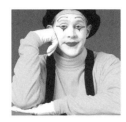

Pause for thought

Look at the plan. When are you reading this book? Has the project been implemented to plan so far?

Look at the plan above and look around you. Is it happening?

If the national programme is to deliver then it has a number of key hurdles to overcome.

• *Technological*: Whilst the system is big, it is not actually revolutionary; the technological issues are all about handling a huge number of transactions.
• *Fitness for clinical purpose*: The solution must demonstrably meet the needs of its users, the clinicians and their patients.
• *Equipping and enthusing clinicians*: There is a need to both train and enthuse clinical staff. Without this it is just a huge empty motorway system with no cars driving around on it.

The key to an effective solution is a whole set of standards, to which the users and developers must adhere.

- *Clinical coding standards*: The information must be stored in the same way across the whole system or the components will not understand information from another part of the system – much like an English person abroad.
- *Data standards*: The data which contain the information must be transmitted in a common format so that each system can extract the information it needs.
- *Network standards*: The links between the systems must be built to common standards, or the transmissions will not work. The whole Internet across the world uses the same network standards or protocols so that all machines can talk to each other. The Internet network protocol is known as TCP/IP.

The latter provides the evidence that the task can be achieved. The Internet is global in scope. It has the potential to link the entire world because everyone agrees to use the same standards. Hopefully the NHS can do the same.

Conclusions

Joined-up information to support joined-up care is a key objective for the NHS. If it can be achieved, it will make clinicians' lives easier, reduce duplicate entry, improve the information available to clinicians to make decisions, speed up care and reduce errors.

The IT people are working very hard to try to make it happen through the National Programme for IT.

Hopefully, they will listen to the clinicians and other NHS staff and provide systems that are fit for purpose and deliver the promised benefits.

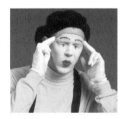

Key points from this chapter

- Patients see the NHS as one organisation: we know different!
- Information transfer between organisations to follow patients is currently problematic.
- The future viability of the NHS depends upon working smarter, including using IT (or so the guru driving government policy believes!).
- The National Programme for IT is currently trying to deliver joined-up IT for the NHS.

5 Informatics can empower patients

The patients – remember them?

Most NHS staff are not in it for the money; they do the job because they care about their patients. We have already seen how information technology can prevent harm to patients and improve their care, especially in the area of health promotion. However, we can go further and use technology to actually give patients more responsibility for their own care and decisions. We shall consider two key areas:

- facilitating self-management
- informing patient decisions.

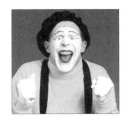

Smile !

Apparently, the jargon word for a patient who arrives at a consultation waving an Internet printout is 'cyberchondriac'.

Facilitating self-management

IT has the potential to allow patients to monitor their own symptoms or conditions in their own homes. This offers a range of potential benefits:

- giving patients more control and ownership over their own health
- allowing more frequent and convenient monitoring
- providing more accurate results in cases where results could be distorted by anxiety, e.g. blood pressure
- accurate recording by electronic transmission into the patient's electronic record
- optional remote monitoring by a clinician and/or warning messages sent to the clinician's desk.

This technology has often been first employed in remote areas, where patients may be a great distance from their clinicians. For example, in Australia this ‘technology has been used in a range of conditions. Typical applications include the management of chronic heart failure (CHF), asthma, diabetes and hypertension. The remote monitoring applications may be supplemented by videophone systems, which allow nurses or doctors to view and talk to the patient while collecting data from equipment that records vital signs.

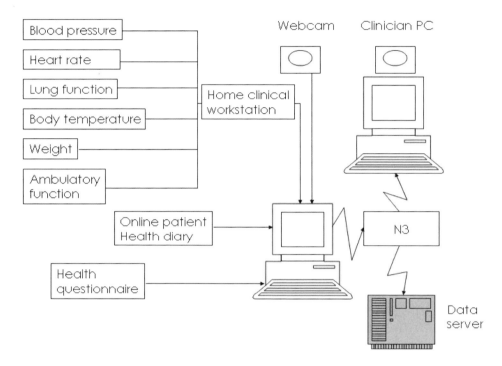

Figure 5.1 Remote monitoring system (adapted from Celler BG, *et al.* Using information technology to improve the management of chronic disease. *MJA* 2003; 179: 242–6. © Copyright 2003. *The Medical Journal of Australia*, reproduced with permission).

The Australian authors carried out a clinical trial.

A clinical trial was carried out over at least 3 months in metropolitan Sydney and in Wagga Wagga (a regional centre) with 22 patients aged 58–82 years. All patients had a primary diagnosis of chronic heart failure and/or chronic obstructive pulmonary disease. Some patients were monitored continuously for more than 8 months.

The Home Telecare System was set up in the patients' homes.

A preliminary patient survey administered before monitoring commenced revealed that the majority of patients had no computer or Internet experience, indeed with 38% having not even used an ATM machine. Visits by the doctor had occurred in 50% of the respondents, with 25% receiving regular visits. A community nurse visited 38% of patients.

A 'Patient's Perceptions' questionnaire demonstrated that patients generally have a high confidence that use of the Home Telecare System will assist with the management of their condition and only have minor concerns over issues of confidentiality and data security (the use of the home telecare technology threatens the confidentiality of my health information, 2.9/6.0).

All patients, despite having almost no prior computer experience, were able to use the system effectively with less than 1 hour of training.

In summary:

- All patients found the Home Telecare System easy to use
- 21 of the 22 patients used the system at least once a day
- 21 of the 22 patients were satisfied with it
- 21 of the 22 patients wanted to continue using the system on a regular basis
- 13 of the 14 GPs who responded stated that they were either very satisfied or satisfied with the system; none expressed dissatisfaction with it.

The article goes on to describe the experience of a 58-year-old female patient with smoking-related chronic obstructive pulmonary disease (COPD) who took part in the trial. The system was used to monitor her lung function, temperature, heart rhythm, weight and blood pressure and these data were reviewed regularly by her general practitioner. The results are shown in Figure 5.2.

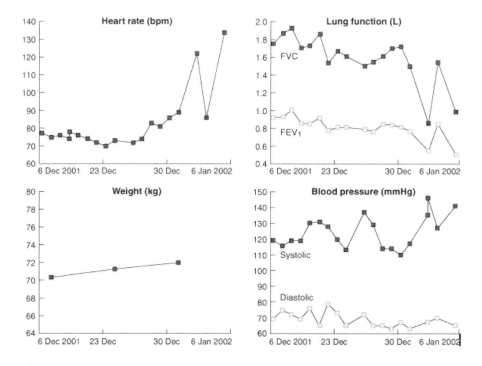

Figure 5.2 Sample results from the monitoring

By monitoring the patient, the GP was able to detect a deterioration in her condition, demonstrated by the development of sinus tachycardia, decreasing forced expiratory volume in one second (FEV1) and forced vital capacity (FVC), and increased weight (presumably due to fluid retention) (see graphs).

In response to the observed data, the GP was able to contact the patient who reported that she was very short of breath. The GP arranged for her to be admitted directly to hospital. At the hospital, the patient was diagnosed with lung infection and mild heart failure. She was discharged after two days of treatment.

It is worth noting that this trial was held in metropolitan Sydney and the town of Wagga Wagga, rather than in the rural outback. The benefits cited would apply to patients in other locations.

However, many of the potential benefits for patients do not need more than access to the Internet.

Informing patient decisions: beyond paternalism

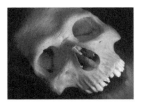

Zombie Warning!

Many clinicians seem to cling to the idea that patients are incapable of making decisions about their own health.

Some may argue that current trends in obesity provide evidence for this zombie: studies on the lifestyles of healthcare professionals suggest that the general public may be no worse than clinicians in this regard.

Current government policy since Wanless II has emphasised the need for patients to take responsibility for their own decisions in relation to a wide range of areas.

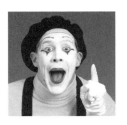

Tip

Wanless II is the second report on the long-term sustainability of the NHS commissioned by the Treasury.

It focuses upon health promotion and education.

It may be accessed in the author's virtual library at:

www.healthlibrary.org.uk

A couple of years ago I was asked to develop an electronic resource to teach people how to find and evaluate health resources on the Internet. The project was funded from resources aimed at patients. However, many of the clinicians felt that it was too dangerous to give such resources directly to patients and the final resources were mediated through clinicians who controlled access to the resources.

A couple of years later, an enhanced resource was developed for ADITUS, the northwest of England NHS Library service, and placed on the public portal.

As with many areas, the clinician's role has changed over the years from being an expert and unchallengeable authority to one whose job is now to guide the patient to the best informed decision. Part of this is the ability to advise patients where to look for resources and how to judge whether they are likely to prove reliable.

Many media organisations have invested in online health resources. Generally, reliable information may be found on websites run by the BBC and the major quality newspapers. This is often a better way for patients to be guided than simply to type their disease name into Google. Other useful resources to which patients may be pointed are sites like Patient UK, which provide details of support groups and patient information leaflets.

NHS sites such as the 'Hitting the Headlines' section of the National Library for Health or NHS Direct Online provide reliable destinations to encourage your patients to visit.

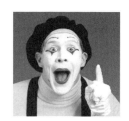

Tip

Faced with the printout-wielding patient or 'cyberchondriac', it is tempting to take the view that the Internet is the spawn of the Devil.

However, a better strategy may be to offer more reliable Internet sites for the patient to visit; many patients will be intending to return to the Internet again, so guidance like this may prevent a return visit to a rogue or inappropriate site.

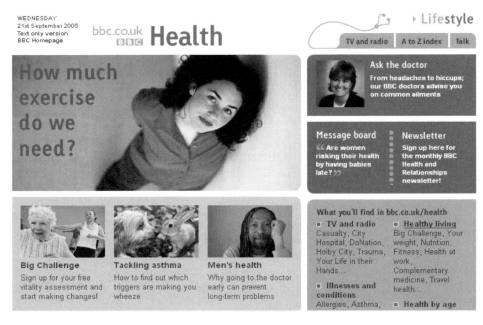

Figure 5.3 The Health section of the BBC website

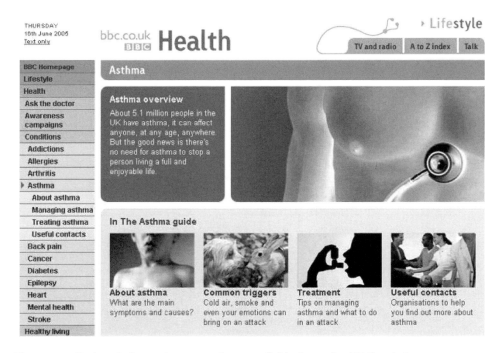

Figure 5.4 Patient information on asthma available from the BBC website

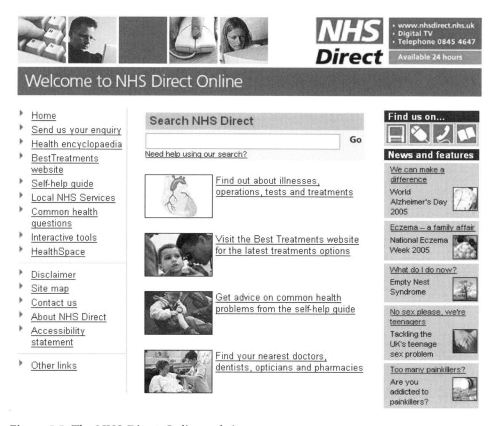

Figure 5.5 The NHS Direct Online website

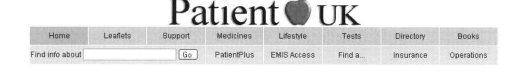

* 681 leaflets on health and disease, some of which have been translated. Most GPs in the UK use these same leaflets to print out for patients and carers during consultations.
* Details of 1971 patient support / self help groups and similar organisations.
* Comprehensive information about medicines and online pharmacy.
* Advice on leading a healthy lifestyle, health promotion and preventing illness.
* Explanations and information about tests and investigations commonly performed.
* A directory of UK websites on disease, health news, events, equipment, helplines, benefits, NHS information, carers' issues, dictionaries, women's health, evidence based medicine, etc.
* Recommended books on health and disease mainly written by UK authors.
* Links to PatientPlus records - quick reference articles used by UK medical professionals.
* Patient Experience - real experiences of medical conditions.
* Find a GP, specialist, hospital, dentist, therapist, counsellor, etc.
* Quotes and information about health / medical insurance and other financial products
* Thinking about having an operation done privately? Find the best prices.

Figure 5.6 The Patient UK website

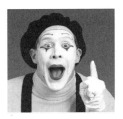

Tip

And for those of you who want to get really up to date, try using the RSS feed on 'Hitting the Headlines' in NLH.

For those of you who feel that you've had quite enough technology, you can skip to the end of the chapter.

The idea of 'Hitting the Headlines' is to provide you as clinicians with evidence to answer questions on the current media stories. At the time of writing it is:

'Ibuprofen and other commonly used painkillers may increase the risk of heart attack, reported eight newspapers (10 June 2005).'

'Hitting the Headlines' provides you with an evidence-based analysis of the story.

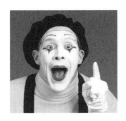

Tip

Although the current story will be different by the time you read this, there is an archive and you should be able to read the full account in the 'Hitting the Headlines' archive. It would be helpful to do so at this point.

The report in 'Hitting the Headlines' starts by linking the media stories to the published study on which the stories were based. It states that:

The reports were accurately based on an observational study that suggested a fairly small absolute increase in risk associated with the prescription of non-steroidal anti-inflammatory drugs (NSAIDs) in primary care.

Hitting the Headlines, 10 June 2005, National Library for Health,
www.nlh.nhs.uk

The report goes on to describe the study and to examine each of the claims made in the media stories. The report concludes with an examination of the underlying evidence for the main conclusion, in this case a link between the use of the drugs and an increased risk of heart attacks.

The report provides information on:

- Where does the evidence come from?
- What were the authors' objectives?
- What was the nature of the evidence?

- How did the participants differ on their levels of exposure to the factor of interest?
- What were the findings?
- What were the authors' conclusions?
- How reliable are the authors' conclusions?
- Are there any systematic reviews on this topic?

Thus the information is designed to help the busy clinician deal with inquiries from anxious patients.

By combining this with the RSS technology, you can provide instant access to this feature on your computer desktop, and it will automatically update to the latest stories.

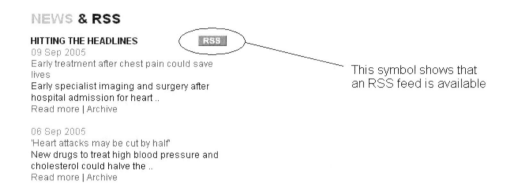

Figure 5.7 The RSS feed from the National Library for Health

The way to access an RSS (Really Simple Syndication) varies according to your reader software. I use the active bookmark feature of my Firefox browser, and add the link to the RSS feed to my bookmark toolbar, which appears just below the main toolbar. The net result is instant access to the evidence behind the latest media stories.

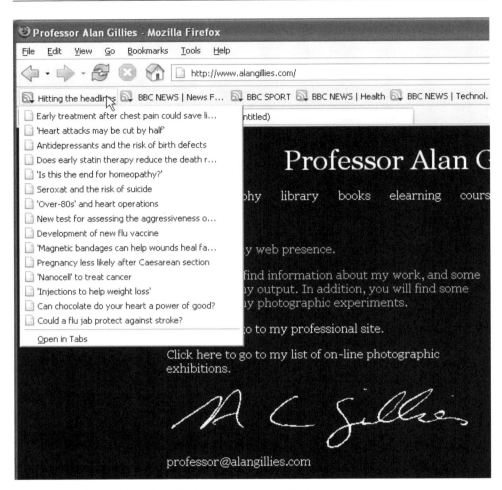

Figure 5.8 The RSS feed installed on the author's desktop

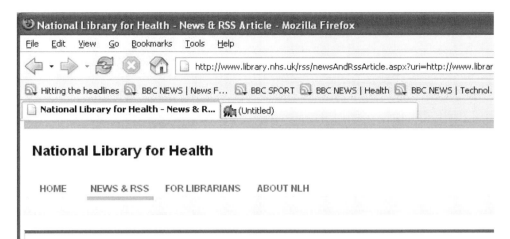

Figure 5.9 The latest evidence accessed from the RSS feed menu

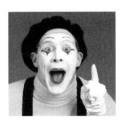

Tip

If there are any Firefox users out there who want detailed instructions on how to achieve this, then email me on professor@alangillies.com

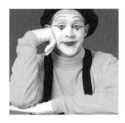

Pause for thought

Have you been faced by cyberchondriacs or even Daily Telegraph-brandishing patients as a result of media scare stories?

If so, visit the National Library for Health next time you're near a computer with Internet access and see if it's in the 'Hitting the Headlines' archive.

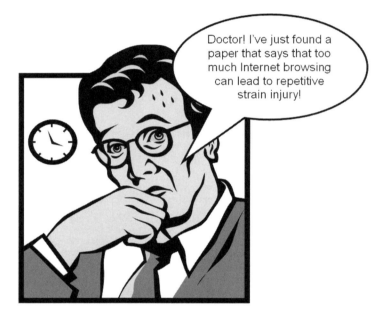

Doctor! I've just found a paper that says that too much Internet browsing can lead to repetitive strain injury!

Figure 5.10 The cyberchondriac

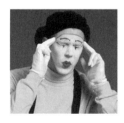

Key points from this chapter

IT can be used to empower patients. We have looked at two applications.

1 IT can be used to monitor a patient remotely in their own home, giving them greater ownership of their own care.
2 IT can be used to provide information for patients to help them make informed decisions.

Part II

What do I need to do for informatics?

6 Be professional

Your professional responsibilities

The basic tenets of any treatment of professional responsibilities are the classical ethical principles of beneficence and non-maleficence. Put simply, beneficence is about doing good, and non-maleficence is about not doing harm.

Throughout this book, we are trying to show that information is a powerful tool for good or bad, and an increasingly important part of patient care. Thus, applying these key principles to our use of information is more important than ever. These principles are deeply ingrained in healthcare professionals. Sometimes, when thinking about using IT and the information made available through the technology, we may not see the consequences.

As a practising clinician, you are subject to professional codes of conduct, and a surprising number of them relate to the use of information, and therefore IT. Healthcare professionals have a responsibility to keep their patients safe, and if that is achieved, to do the most good that they can for them.

Until recently, this could be achieved without the benefit of a computer. This is no longer true. Even at the current nascent stage of technology, there are areas where every clinician can improve their practice by the appropriate use of computers.

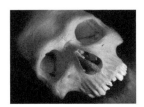

Zombie Warning!

The idea that the use of IT is still not an integral part of routine clinical care still persists.

However, this argument is a zombie. The evidence no longer supports it, although I'm well aware that the view is common.

Increasingly, there are also areas where inappropriate use of IT could harm patients.

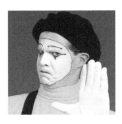

Warning!

Consider the case of a prescription issued in primary care. With over 95% of prescriptions in primary care issued by computer, a doctor who issued a prescription without using available IT facilities, with their inbuilt safeguards, which resulted in an adverse event could, I believe, be prosecuted for negligence, since the legal defence that s/he had done everything that his/her peers would normally have done would not be sustainable.

This means that use of IT by clinicians is subject to the same professional standards as other aspects of clinical care. Many of you who are clinicians will hold this truth to be self-evident. However, in order to make it a universal reality, staff must be competent to deliver the same professional standards while working in unfamiliar ways with unfamiliar technology.

Codes of conduct

In Table 6.1 we consider the 14 duties of a doctor registered with the GMC and their information implications.

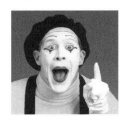

Tip

These duties are taken from the GMC website, where you will find further guidance on a number of key areas, including consent and confidentiality.

Similar standards exist for all healthcare professionals:

As a registered nurse, midwife or specialist community public health nurse, you are personally accountable for your practice. In caring for patients and clients, you must:

- respect the patient or client as an individual
- obtain consent before you give any treatment or care
- protect confidential information
- co-operate with others in the team
- maintain your professional knowledge and competence
- be trustworthy
- act to identify and minimise risk to patients and clients.

NMC *Code of Conduct*, 2004a

Table 6.1 The implications for information handling of the 14 duties of a doctor registered with the GMC

1 make the care of your patient your first concern	This suggests a requirement to make use of all available resources to ensure that patients receive the best possible care, including accessing evidence, using decision support and keeping high-quality records
2 treat every patient politely and considerately	This does not require IT, but suggests a need for sensitivity to ensure that the technology does not intrude unduly into a consultation
3 respect patients' dignity and privacy	This is at the heart of the clinician's responsibilities towards consent, confidentiality and data security
4 listen to patients and respect their views	IT provides new ways of communicating with patients and an opportunity to improve two-way communication
5 give patients information in a way they can understand	Again, IT provides new ways of communicating with patients and providing new types of information, for example, graphical, animated and video information
6 respect the rights of patients to be fully involved in decisions about their care	IT allows patients access to a much greater range of sources of information; some of these may be incorrect or even dangerous, therefore clinicians have a responsibility to guide patients to appropriate resources and away from inappropriate resources
7 keep your professional knowledge and skills up to date	IT allows clinicians access to a much greater range of sources of information as well. To not take advantage of this could be regarded as negligent
8 recognise the limits of your professional competence	This applies just as much to competence in handling information and IT as to clinical competencies
9 be honest and trustworthy	The only implication here is to ensure that clinicians apply the same standards to handling information as they do in all other aspects of clinical practice
10 respect and protect confidential information	To do this using an IT system may seem more complicated than with a paper-based system. The fundamental principle remains and should be honoured

Table 6.1 (*cont.*)

11 make sure that your personal beliefs do not prejudice your patients' care	You may believe that IT is the invention of the Devil: however, you have a responsibility to take a more balanced view!
12 act quickly to protect patients from risk if you have good reason to believe that you or a colleague may not be fit to practise	IT does facilitate many aspects of performance management, and allow you to investigate any concerns you may have. On the other hand, information is no more or less valid because it is stored on a computer, and should always be interpreted with care!
13 avoid abusing your position as a doctor	The only implication here is to ensure that clinicians apply the same standards to handling information as they do in all other aspects of clinical practice
14 work with colleagues in the ways that best serve patients' interests	There are many implications here about using technology to share information across a multiprofessional team. There is a responsibility to make use of the technology to facilitate joined-up working in the interests of the patient, but also issues over consent to information sharing, confidentiality and security.

The Nursing and Midwifery Council has produced detailed guidance on record keeping, available from the NMC website:

> The Nursing and Midwifery Council (NMC) believes that record keeping is a fundamental part of nursing, midwifery and specialist community public health nursing practice.
>
> NMC, 2004b

The guidance has the following specific advice on electronic patient records:

> Many registered nurses, midwives and specialist community public health nurses regularly use information technology to record the planning, assessment and delivery of care. There are obvious advantages to this.
>
> Computer-held records tend to be easier to read, less bulky, reduce the need for duplication and can increase communication across the inter-professional healthcare team. However, the same basic principles that apply to manual records must be applied to computer-held records. You do not need to keep manual duplicates of computer-held records and they do not replace the need to maintain dialogue throughout the inter-professional healthcare team. Safeguards for computer-held records must be in compliance with the Computer Misuse Act 1990.

Security, access and confidentiality

The principle of the confidentiality of information held about your patients and clients is just as important in computer-held records as in all other records, including those sent by fax. You are professionally accountable for making sure that whatever system is used is fully secure. Clear local protocols should be drawn up to specify which staff have access to computer-held records. Although patients and clients can expect their health records to be accessed by different members of the inter-professional healthcare team, this should only be done where necessary.

Patients and clients do not have the right to limit the amount of information relevant to their care or condition that is incorporated in their records. However, they can limit access to certain information about themselves and you must respect their right to do so. Local guidelines and protocols should address this right and these procedures should also include ways of establishing the date and time of any entry, the person who made the entry, and should ensure that any changes or additions to entries are made in such a way that the original information is still visible and accessible.

Accountability and computer-held records

You are accountable for any entry you make to a computer-held record and you must ensure that any entry you make is clearly identifiable.

NMC, 2004*

Record keeping

One of the most important areas of change is in the nature of record keeping. In primary care, a significant amount of recording has been done directly onto computer records for a number of years. However, in other areas of the health service, clinicians have not been in direct contact with computerised clinical records.

This is a profound change, and we may expect resistance. A few years ago, I was visiting an outpatient clinic as a patient. Not wanting to miss an opportunity, I called in on the IT department beforehand and discussed their planned deployment of an electronic patient records system.

'Are the clinicians on board?' I asked.

'Oh yes!' I was assured.

Thirty minutes later I was conversing as readily as it is possible to do with a large uncomfortable tube up my nasal passages:

'I hear that you're getting a new computerised patient records system.'

'They'd better not bring it anywhere near me!'

It is important to recognise that IT is about enabling new ways of working, and often it is those new ways of working that cause the problems rather than the technology itself.

For example, in order to establish proper audit trails, every entry on the record will be linked to a specific person. Their access rights will depend upon their status and need to know information. This raises the possibility of consultants being issued with personalised access cards linked to them by biometric details to maximise security, and only they being allowed to enter clinical data onto the record.

This requires a major shift away from the current situation where recording of information is likely to be split between the consultant's secretary and specialist coders.

There is already evidence that in some locations, frustration or inadequate skills are leading clinicians to omit information from clinical records or to input inaccurate information, in direct contradiction of their professional codes of conduct shown above.

New consultation skills

Consider the following situation.

A 15-year-old girl comes to see you, as her clinician. She wishes to receive the contraceptive pill as she is embarking on a sexual relationship with her boyfriend. She does not wish you to inform her parents of this. After encouraging her to speak to her parents and carrying out all the appropriate health checks, you agree to prescribe the pill, and enter the prescription into her electronic health record.

Three weeks later, she returns to the surgery with her mother for treatment for a minor unrelated condition.

The use of electronic records raises some new issues around confidentiality. In general, it is a good idea to encourage the patient to view their record with you in a consultation. However, in this case, this needs careful handling to maintain confidentiality regarding the previous consultation.

A further issue may arise if you try to prescribe a medication which is contraindicated by the contraceptive pill. A flashing message on the screen saying that the pill has been prescribed recently may not be helpful!

IT is about facilitating new ways of working. A consultation based around an electronic health record requires new skills – not just IT skills but new types of consultation skill based around the use of the computer within the consultation.

The Department of Health has commissioned research on the impact of IT within the consulting room in general practice. Some of the key findings were as follows:

Common to all the doctors, however, was the desire to minimise the amount of data entry while the patient was in the consulting room. Most were seen to be inputting data after a patient had left the room, while the next patient's record was consulted briefly before they came in. The paper notes, however, were sometimes brought in by the patient and therefore could only be consulted by the doctor during the consultation.

There were also examples of doctors using the computer and the paper notes at the same time – using the paper notes to inform the computer

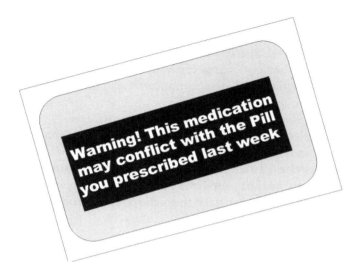

Figure 6.1 Warnings may not help maintain confidentiality

record or vice versa. This was particularly noticeable in the early stages of the consultation where the doctor is 'information gathering'. He may ask the patient a question and while the patient is answering, confirm the information by consulting the computer and the paper records.

From studying the sample of consultations it became clear that there was not going to be one template that could describe the ultimate way to manage the computer within the consultation. It appeared that individual doctors found a variety of ways of minimising the impact of the computer. From the research a number of general behaviours were identified to describe the different ways doctors approached computer use and secondly a number of strategies were also identified, which were employed by doctors to prevent the computer interfering with the rapport between doctor and patient.

Position of the computer screen

Behaviour and attitude to the computer may be influenced or aided by the position of the computer within the consulting room in relation to the doctor and the patient (although it must be stressed that an exact correlation was not identified). Of course, not all doctors will have a choice about the position of the computer, due to the physical restraints of the room layout or the fact that they share the room with other doctors.

Three main positions were identified

1 The doctor has the screen and keyboard on the desk immediately in front of him. He sits at an angle of 45 degrees to the screen to face the patient, but can turn his head and type or search for information on the screen, without having to turn his body away from the patient. The position of the computer allows for opportunistic computer use (for example, the doctor can glance at the screen while the patient is rolling up their sleeve or taking

off their coat). The doctor can glance surreptitiously at the screen even while talking to the patient, without the patient really noticing. If he needs to change the screen, the doctor can tap the keys with his left hand and again, he doesn't need to change his body posture. Doctors who use paper notes in conjunction with the computer may prefer to have a space in front of them on the desk to place the notes. For this reason, some doctors may place the computer to one side or other of centre.

2 The screen is placed on the desk mid-way between patient and doctor. This position is conducive to the sharing of electronic information between doctor and patient. The screen faces squarely into the room and can be seen by the patient from their seat (some doctors may have the screen facing slightly towards them and actually turn the screen round to face the patient when they want to show information on the screen). Having the computer between doctor and patient allows the patient to read the screen while the doctor is using it or to read a shared screen with the doctor.

This raises the issues around patient confidentiality. For example, sensitive information on the screen can be accidentally read by a spouse or relative who has come into the consultation with the patient. The doctor can avoid this by turning the screen away from the patient but it can lead to an awkward moment.

Similarly, if patients are to share information on the electronic record, is there information that is not suitable for them to see? What counts as suitable information? Does a patient have a right to see their own record? Could information viewed be damaging, upsetting, misread or taken out of context? What may be upsetting to one patient may not be to another and so how is this gauged? As we move away from the paternalistic model of the doctor towards the patient as consumer with more control over their healthcare, all these issues become problematic. The computer has a part to play in the shift away from the doctor as the fount of all knowledge. Sharing information on the screen with the patient is moving away from 'let me tell you what is wrong with you' to 'let's look on the computer and see if we can find out'.

3 The screen is placed away from the patient on the other side of the doctor. This necessitates the doctor swinging round in his chair and virtually turning his back on the patient while he attends to the screen. This position could lead to the doctor seeming to ignore the patient. The computer on the opposite side of the desk to the patient can also be conducive to controlling the consultation, as if the doctor turns away and begins to type, this gives a clear message that the doctor is engaged in the computer and eye contact has been lost. Often if the doctor turns overtly away from the patient to the screen, the patient is seen to:
- raise their voice as they are talking and /or
- lean forward towards the doctor and /or
- allow their sentence to trail off as they are not sure whether the doctor is listening, or whether it is OK to interrupt the task.

When the computer was placed in this position, sometimes, not only did the doctor turn away from the patient to attend to the screen, but also he actually slid his chair away from the patient, a further reason why rapport could be lost. Once the doctor had finished on the computer, he would slide his chair back towards the patient.

There was considerable crossover between the position of the computer and models of computer use adopted, but position of the screen could arguably facilitate some methods more than others.

Printer use

Finally, the impact of the printer upon the consultation was also considered. Whilst printing off prescriptions, at the end of the consultation, a significant amount of noise is generated (possibly exaggerated on the video recordings). Could this noise drown out the patient who may be saying something significant to the doctor? One general observation made was that the noise of the printer often signified the end of the consultation, as the noise often appeared to drown out speech. It also necessitates the doctor's attention firstly upon the screen and keyboard as he types a prescription and then upon the printer to tear off the necessary paper. Often the doctor had to stand and/or turn his back on the patient to do this. The printer noise often provided a non-verbal signal that the consultation has reached a close, as is the doctor's pre-occupation with the printer. This was often a cue for the patient to stand up and put on their coat. Some doctors attempted to maintain rapport while the computer was printing. On one occasion, the doctor chatted generally about the mist that morning while the printer noise was evident.

Categories of doctor behaviour

Three main categories were identified that describe the behaviour of our sample of doctors within the consultation.

- CONTROLLING – taking control of the consultation from the patient to the doctor, so that the doctor can attend to the computer. An example of this kind of behaviour would be the doctor who turns away from the patient and types in silence. The doctor is indicating that he needs to use the computer, perhaps to move the consultation into another phase.
- RESPONSIVE/OPPORTUNISTIC – these two behaviours can be seen as a continuum. The doctor uses the computer opportunistically, by glancing briefly at the screen so that the patient will hardly notice, or uses the computer while the patent is behind the screen waiting for an examination. At the other end of the scale, the doctor responds to the patient, allowing the patient to lead the consultation times, responding immediately, by refraining from computer use if the patient speaks. The doctor may also include the patient in decision making and share information on the screen.
- IGNORING – the doctor may use the computer in silence and can be seen to ignore or not hear a question or cue from the patient. This behaviour

raises the question of 'can the doctor multi-task?'. In other words can a doctor engage with the computer and also listen fully to a patient who may be talking simultaneously?

These themes and strategies are not mutually exclusive. A doctor may show behaviour covering more than one theme within a consultation and similarly use a variety of strategies to keep the rapport between doctor and patient intact. The types of behaviour identified are not clearly demarcated and can be seen as a range of behaviours on a continuum.

Taken from *IT in the Consulting Room: Final Report,*
July 2002 SCHIN/DoH*

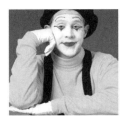

Pause for thought

If you work in a consulting room or area with a computer screen on your desk then think about the following.

- How is the room arranged?
- How do you behave towards the computer and patient?
- Are you controlling, responsive or ignoring?
- If you have no computer in your treatment area, where would you put it?

What do I need to know?

From this chapter, it should be obvious that if clinicians are to operate as effective professionals, they will need to learn new skills in order to work in the new ways offered by the IT. The skills needed go beyond the IT skills to include all the skills to use the technology within a different way of working.

We may like to think of three categories of skills needed.

1 *IT skills*: These are the basic skills needed to operate the technology.
2 *Adaptive skills*: These are the areas where clinicians have existing skills, e.g. confidentiality, consultation, which may need to be changed or enhanced to work in new ways with IT.
3 *New non-IT skills*: In some cases, entirely new skills are needed that are not technology related. For example, it is likely that most clinicians will need some understanding and skills in the area of coding, which their current role may not need.

Skills for Health, working with the NHS Information Centre for Health and Social Care, has recently defined national occupational standards for clinical informatics, which go some way to addressing these issues. These standards are still in draft at the time of writing: however, eight competences have been identified and defined.

HI 120   Identify the needs of clinicians, patients and the public for communication, information and knowledge systems

HI 121   Develop a specification for communication, information and knowledge systems to meet the needs of clinicians, patients and the public

HI 122   Facilitate, and clinically validate, the development of communication, information and knowledge systems to meet the needs of an agreed specification

HI 123   Facilitate, and clinically validate, the implementation, evaluation and improvement of communication, information and knowledge systems to meet the needs of clinicians, patients and the public

HI 124   Facilitate the clinical audit process

HI 125   Search for clinical information and evidence according to an accepted methodology

HI 126   Critically appraise clinical information and evidence

HI 127   Develop evidence-based clinical guidelines

Here is the full draft specification for the first of the standards.

National Occupational Standards for Clinical Informatics*

HI 120 Identify the needs of clinicians, patients and the public for communication, information and knowledge systems

About this competence

This competence is about identifying the needs of clinicians, patients and the public for communication, information and knowledge systems. It is relevant to individuals who are working with a variety of stakeholders to develop the clinical application of communication, information and knowledge systems.

Links

To be completed.

Origin

This is a new competence developed by Skills for Health.

Key words and concepts

Communication, information and knowledge systems

The work processes, and communication, information and knowledge systems and services that are used to directly support the delivery of care that is based on the best available evidence.

Scope

Dialogue concerning the care process

The dialogue concerning the care process may include:

a what is done
b how it is done
c why it is done
d who does it
e any potential improvements

Needs

Needs:

a for information to support the delivery of care
b of systems to support the delivery of care

Recommendations

Recommendations may include:

a improvements based on systems
b improvements to work processes
c no change

Stakeholders

Stakeholders may include:

a patients
b clinicians
c the public
d other professions (including IT staff)
e allied workers (e.g. estates)
f suppliers
g managers
h carers

Performance criteria

You need to:

1 identify the stakeholders that need to be involved in relation to the communication, information and knowledge systems you are concerned with
2 identify the appropriate processes to use for involving stakeholders
3 conduct a dialogue concerning the care process with stakeholders to help inform the development of communication, information and knowledge systems
4 discuss the potential benefits and challenges of the clinical application of communication, information and knowledge systems with stakeholders
5 manage expectations effectively throughout the process

6 identify the needs of stakeholders for communication, information and knowledge systems based on their involvement

7 fully consider the risks of the clinical application of communication, information and knowledge systems

8 clearly document the outcomes of the work and make appropriate recommendations

Knowledge and understanding

You need to apply:

Legal and organisational

1 working knowledge of the wider political sensitivities of data, information and knowledge

2 working knowledge of current legislation, policies, procedures, codes of practice and guidelines in relation to the clinical application of communication, information and knowledge systems

3 working knowledge of the professional codes of ethics relevant to the areas of your work, including those of other professions you are working with

4 working knowledge of the health context for data, information and knowledge requirements (e.g. clinical impact, patient safety)

5 working knowledge of your organisation's planning cycles and objectives

6 working knowledge of the care delivery process in the area of work you are focusing your attention on

7 in-depth understanding of the importance and reasons for adhering to information governance including: confidentiality, consent, data protection, security and privacy

8 in-depth understanding of the different ways in which data, information and knowledge are used in healthcare

Communication, information and knowledge systems

9 working knowledge of the communication, information and knowledge systems in your organisation

10 working knowledge of the current developments in the clinical application of communication, information and knowledge systems relevant to the areas of your work

11 working knowledge of the staff responsible for maintaining and developing the technical aspects of communication, information and knowledge systems and their ways of working

12 in-depth understanding of the ways in which clinicians and other users interact with communication, information and knowledge systems (i.e. identified roles and responsibilities)

13 in-depth understanding of the reasons why there are limitations to what can be achieved with communication, information and knowledge

systems

14 in-depth understanding of local coding practice and data definitions that exist and how this impacts on data migration

15 critical understanding of the risks in relation to the clinical application of communication, information and knowledge systems

Stakeholder involvement

16 in-depth understanding of the clinical needs of the stakeholders that will use the communication, information and knowledge systems

17 in-depth understanding of the range of stakeholders that will require an input to your work on communication, information and knowledge systems

18 in-depth understanding of how to identify the stakeholders to involve

19 in-depth understanding of how to involve stakeholders with communication, information and knowledge systems and the processes you can use for this

20 in-depth understanding of how to interpret the needs and manage expectations of stakeholders

21 critical understanding of the processes for documenting the outcomes of the work and making recommendations

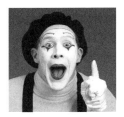

Tip

The full standards are available on the web.

Try the Information Centre website for full details. www.ic.nhs.uk

Particularly good as a cure for insomnia: that's standards for you – boring but important.

Increasingly, within the NHS, job specifications and remuneration are being linked to these standards, and so they will become increasingly important over the coming years.

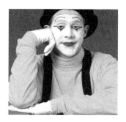

Pause for thought

If you have access to the Internet, track down the standards: if not, or if you have problems, ask your NHS librarian to help you access them.

How many of the competency items do you currently feel able to meet?

How many of the competency items don't feel relevant to you?

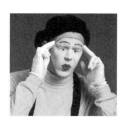

Key points from this chapter

- IT is now a core part of professional clinical practice.
- IT changes the way in which professionals work.
- IT does not change a professional's obligations in terms of their codes of conduct.
- The new ways of working facilitated by IT require professionals to acquire a range of new skills.
- The NOS for clinical informatics are designed to help define what new skills people need.

7 Data standards

Boring but important

Standards are not inherently interesting but they are essential to daily lives. Look around the room you are reading this book in. There are things that depend upon standards all around you. For example, all the electrical appliances need to receive electrical power of a certain voltage and frequency.

If there is a television in the room, then there are many different standards needed to ensure that every television can receive every broadcast and show it correctly. The same goes for a radio, a CD, a DVD player and so on . . .

If our NHS information systems were railways, then the trains would fall off the tracks; if they were CDs, they would not play on your machines. So how do we build information systems that can talk to each other? For this we need a layer cake, a seven-layer cake!

The bits someone else will worry about

In order for computer systems to talk to each other, we need to establish common standards for communications. These ensure that the infrastructure works. Think of it as like the standards that ensure your television works, or your electricity. If they weren't there, you'd notice. But we expect the electricity to be there, the television to work and the rails on the railways to be the same distance apart. Generally they are! So we don't have to worry about those.

The bits you have to worry about

However, there are some bits that you do have to worry about.

You may well have heard the expression 'garbage in, garbage out', meaning that computers are only as good as the data they are given. But I'm afraid it's worse than that: you see, computers are stupid – it's not their fault, it's the way they are made.

The reasoning goes something like this. When we describe something we use natural language. We communicate with words, but they are ambiguous. It has been calculated that, on average, most words in the English language have four distinct meanings and this is too much for the poor computers. They need everything to be black and white. They have to be able to reduce everything to ones and zeros ultimately. So, for example, you might use the word 'heart' to mean:

- the organ that pumps blood
- the essence of the matter
- courage or spirit.

This would leave a computer thoroughly confused. And it works the other way, too. A doctor might talk about a myocardial infarction, a patient about a heart attack. Unless you tell the computer, it doesn't know that these are the same thing.

This is the reason why we have to use codes to describe diagnoses, drugs, treatments, etc. for the computer – to tell it precisely what we mean. This may help the computer, but it leaves us with three distinct problems.

1 We have to make sure that everyone is using the same coding system.
2 We have to make sure everyone is using the same codes for the same things.
3 The real world is ambiguous, and this is why clever humans have developed ways of handling ambiguity. The poor stupid computer has not.

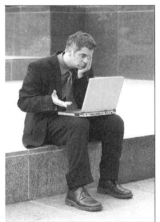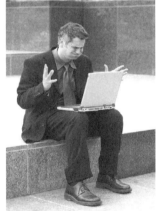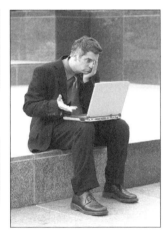

Figure 7.1 Computers ARE stupid: it's not their fault – it's the way they are made

Computers need their information in a particular form. When it all boils down to it, a computer's brain is just a collection of light switches that are on or off. This means that what may make perfect sense to you appears to the computer as complete rubbish. Even the slowest human brain by comparison is capable of all sorts of interpretative tasks that computers don't have a clue about.

So if I wrote 'astma' on the record of a child whose mother had brought them to see you because they were wheezing, you would assume that I meant 'asthma' and I couldn't spell. The computer would look at 'astma' and say, THIS IS NOT ASTHMA. True, but unhelpful.

But once we operate in the computer's world, the roles are reversed. If six clinicians coded 'asthma' on a child's electronic record, they might use different codes to reflect subtleties about the condition; the computer sees six codes, six conditions. Unless we specifically tell the computer that each code represents the same thing, then it will assume that they are different. It will only search for the specific codes that you tell it to. Therefore, you must make sure that those are the same codes that were used to store the data.

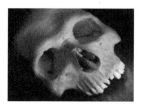

Zombie Warning!

There is a common view that 'to err is human, but to really screw up takes a computer'.

Although computers are stupid, they don't make mistakes within their operating limits. So while computers are convenient scapegoats, this view fits my definition of an intellectual zombie.

Let's consider this a bit further.

In order to get seven quality points under the 2004 GMS Contract and the funding that follows, practices need to be able to produce a register of patients with asthma, excluding patients with asthma who have been prescribed no asthma-related drugs in the last 12 months (7 points). In order to find the patients with asthma, the computer needs to look for:

- H33 Asthma
- H33.11 Bronchial asthma
- H330 Extrinsic (atopic) asthma
- H330.11 Allergic asthma
- H330.12 Childhood asthma
- H330.13 Hay fever with asthma
- H330.14 Pollen asthma
- H3300 Extrinsic asthma without status asthmaticus
- H330011 Hay fever with asthma
- H3301 Extrinsic asthma with status asthmaticus
- H330111 Extrinsic asthma with asthma attack
- H330z Extrinsic asthma NOS
- H331 Intrinsic asthma
- H331.11 Late-onset asthma
- H3310 Intrinsic asthma without status asthmaticus
- H3311 Intrinsic asthma with status asthmaticus
- H331111 Intrinsic asthma with asthma attack
- H331z Intrinsic asthma NOS
- H332 Mixed asthma
- H333 Acute exacerbation of asthma
- H33z Asthma unspecified
- H33z0 Status asthmaticus NOS
- H33z011 Severe asthma attack

- H33z1 Asthma attack
- H33z111 Asthma attack NOS
- H33z2 Late-onset asthma
- H33zz Asthma NOS
- H33zz11 Exercise-induced asthma
- H33zz12 Allergic asthma NEC
- H33zz13 Allergic bronchitis NEC

In addition it needs to find patients that are excluded from monitoring, coded as:

- 9hA1 Excepted from asthma quality indicators: Patient unsuitable
- 9hA2 Excepted from asthma quality indicators: Informed dissent
- 9OJ2 Refuses asthma monitoring

Actually, finding the codes is easy: you can simply add a query that someone else has written to do this for you. But the query will only find those patients who have been correctly coded, or the poor limited computer won't know.

For example, in order to meet the requirements of the 2004 GMS Contract, and gain the quality points for asthmas, the codes entered must precisely match the criteria:

Indicator	Description	Read Code narrative	Codes
ASTHMA 1 7 points	Patients with asthma excluding patients with asthma who have been prescribed no asthma-related drugs in the last 12 months	Asthma SELECTIVE BETA-ADRENOCEPTOR STIMULANT Except **SALINE FOR NEBULISATION** ANTICHOLINERGIC BRONCHODILATORS XANTHINE BRONCHODILATORS Except **CAFFEINE** COMPOUND BRONCHODILATORS CORTICOSTEROIDS [RESPIRATORY USE] ASTHMA PROPHYLAXIS LEUKOTRIENE RECEPTOR ANTAGONIST	H33% c1% c1A.. c3% c4% c44.. c5% c6% c7% cA%

What type of problems are there and how do we spot them?

Data errors come in two principal types:

- data which are impossible
- data which are possible, but incorrect.

Data that cannot be true can be detected by the computer. Examples might include:

- Date of birth: 29/56/1963
- Weight: 12 000 kg
- Post code   1PR HE2

All of these values lie outside the possible values for these fields.

We can use contextual knowledge to look for combinations of data that are impossible. For example, if we find the code 685H on the record of a male patient, it implies that the patient has had a benign hysterectomy, and should therefore be excluded from cervical screening. The reality, of course, is that this is impossible and therefore it is a data error.

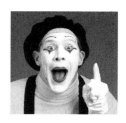

Tip

Spurious male hysterectomies have often been used as a measure of data quality.

Clearly, the fewer found, the better the data!

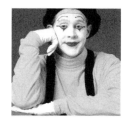

Pause for thought

What other measures might you use, which might be more relevant to your own field?

The second type of error is those that are possible but incorrect in this case, normally arising from typing errors. These are much more difficult to spot, particularly where the incorrect value is perfectly plausible. It is also worth noting that many users will scan the values being input visually. This may well detect an error in an order series of characters, e.g. a word of text, but not in what appears to be an unordered alphanumerical sequence such as a Read Code.

However, IT can help here, this time to try to prevent such errors through good interface design. If we consider the asthma case again, and we wish to enter the code for:

- H330.13 Hay fever with asthma

a good interface will guide us to the correct answer exploiting the hierarchical nature of the Read Code system.

Table 7.1 Example of exploiting the hierarchical nature of the Read Code system

		H330.11 Allergic asthma
H33 Asthma	H330 Extrinsic (atopic) asthma	H330.12 Childhood asthma
	H331 Intrinsic asthma	H330.13 Hay fever with asthma
	H332 Mixed asthma	H330.14 Pollen asthma
	H333 Acute exacerbation of asthma	

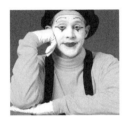

Pause for thought

When people talk about the usability of information systems they normally mean how easy they are to use.

The issue of guiding you away from wrong answers is often not considered.

An extension of this principle is the use of clinical guidelines and protocols that guide clinicians through a standardised process and on the way make sure that the correct standardised codes are entered into the patient record.

For example, in Scotland one local health board has worked with practices to implement a standard guideline for epilepsy (*see* Figure 7.2). Not only can the computer system guide the clinician through the process, but it can enter the standard codes on the record as the process progresses, or offer the clinician an appropriate set of codes from which they can select an option.

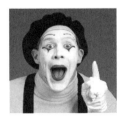

Tip

Within primary care, the PRIMIS project has been operating for a number of years with considerable success in boosting data quality through a combination of facilitation, training and resources.

Visit the PRIMIS website for more information: www.primis.nhs.uk

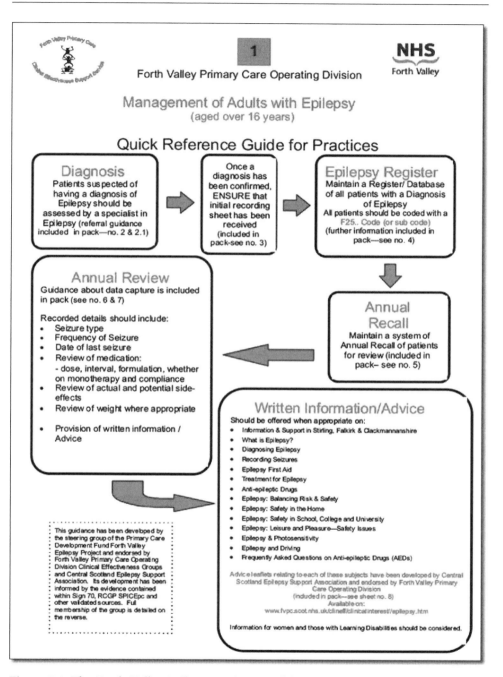

Figure 7.2 The Forth Valley Epilepsy Project Guideline

SNOMED: the future (?)

Part of the fragmentation of the NHS has been the use of a range of coding schema. Read Code has achieved primacy in primary care, but has not been adopted in other sectors. Even Read Codes come in a range of versions.

In an attempt to provide a common coding standard, the NHS has got together with the College of American Pathologists to define a new common coding language called SNOMED CT, based upon Read Codes and SNOMED.

> SNOMED Clinical Terms (SNOMED CT) is a dynamic, scientifically validated clinical healthcare terminology and infrastructure that makes healthcare knowledge more usable and accessible. The SNOMED CT core terminology provides a common language that enables a consistent way of capturing, sharing and aggregating health data across specialties and sites of care. Among the applications for SNOMED CT are electronic medical records, ICU monitoring, clinical decision support, medical research studies, clinical trials, computerized physician order entry, disease surveillance, image indexing and consumer health information services.
>
> College of American Pathologists website

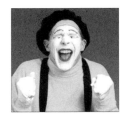

Smile !

Well, they would say that, wouldn't they?

The NHS Connecting for Health programme is a little more cautious in its claims:

> SNOMED CT has been selected as the standard terminology scheme for the National Programme for IT (NPfIT). The use of SNOMED will greatly enhance consistent recording and communication of clinical information. There are challenges in the training of staff and migration from current systems, both of which are being considered by the National Programme.
>
> Implementation questions, 1.4, Connecting for Health website

So just what is SNOMED CT? In 1999 the NHS and the College of American Pathologists (CAP) agreed to merge SNOMED with the NHS Clinical Terms (the Read Codes) to produce a single joint clinical terminology – SNOMED CT (clinical terminology). The merger was completed in 2002 with the first release of SNOMED CT.

While SNOMED has its origins in North American pathology laboratories, the Read Codes were developed during the mid-1980s as a comprehensive coding and classification scheme for British GPs to record almost anything in an electronic patient record.

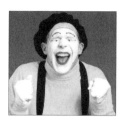

Smile !

My favourite Read Code was always 'Accidental poisoning in an opera house', now sadly obsolete. The one which raised a question in my mind was 'Judicial execution: electric chair'. I've yet to track down a British GP who's had cause to use that one in morning surgery.

Their simple hierarchical structure was based around the organisation of the International Classification of Diseases, the OPCS Classification of Procedures and the British National Formulary for medicines.

In formal terms, SNOMED CT is the dictionary of clinical terms used in clinical communications and electronic healthcare records, including the National Care Records Service.

While in the realms of pedantry, strictly SNOMED CT is both a coding scheme – identifying concepts and terms – and a multidimensional classification, enabling concepts to be related to each other, grouped and analysed according to different criteria. Codes and classifications do different jobs. Codes are unambiguous identifiers of concepts, whereas classifications put instances into categories according to pre-defined criteria. Codes identify, while classifications group for analysis.

SNOMED CT uses numeric codes to identify every instance of its three core building blocks: concepts, descriptions and relationships. Each concept represents a single specific meaning; each description associates a single term with a concept (any concept may have any number of descriptions or names); and each relationship represents a logical relationship between two concepts.

SNOMED CT contains over 300 000 concepts, 1 million descriptions and 1.5 million relationships. In comparison, ICD-10 has 10 760 classes traditionally used by epidemiologists to classify diseases.

SNOMED codes are linked within the dictionary to define relationships between concepts. For example, the concept 'fracture of the tibia' has an explicit relationship with the concept 'tibia', to define the site of fracture. Relationships are also used to build expressions within patient records. For example, the concept of fracture of shaft of tibia can be qualified by laterality (laterality = right) and by fracture type (fracture type = spiral). This is known as post-coordination.

SNOMED CT is only used in computer systems – it cannot be used manually. First, because it is so large, but more importantly because it works in a different way from earlier coding schemes such as ICD or the Read Codes. In these schemes the relationship between concepts is specified within the code itself. For example, in ICD-10, the code for fracture of shaft of tibia is S82.2, which is a specialisation of S82 (fracture of lower leg including ankle).

In SNOMED CT this taxonomy (hierarchy) is maintained as separate relationships, which rely on computer software to work. SNOMED CT's relationship mechanism is more complex than a code-dependent hierarchy, but is enormously more powerful and flexible. It allows any concept to be classified or qualified in any number of ways.

Every Read Code ever released is present in SNOMED CT, so migration from Read Codes to SNOMED CT will not result in loss of information. SNOMED CT provides an extensible foundation for expressing clinical data in both local systems and in the National Care Record System within the NPfIT view of the world. However, SNOMED CT is much larger and more complex than any previous coding scheme. The relationship structure is completely different.

However, there remain concerns. Experienced users of Read Codes may not be keen to migrate their data, in view of previous experience where data transfer has led to errors of up to 20%, and it is therefore crucial that the data transfer process is as good as it can be.

In reality, the NPfIT depends on having a common language for gathering and sharing medical knowledge. SNOMED CT will be the language of the NHS Care Records Service and is designed to cut down the potential for differing interpretations of information and the possibility of errors resulting from traditional paper records.

If clinical information is to be transferred and exchanged electronically, a standard clinical terminology is a necessary component of clinical systems. There would be problems in exchange of information for clinical or managerial purposes if several vocabularies and terms for the same topic were used within the NHS. SNOMED CT is, therefore, to be maintained and updated centrally. There will, however, be opportunities to submit requests for terms to be amended or introduced at a 'submission request' area on the NHS Terminology Service website.

It is likely that the use of SNOMED CT will meet less resistance in those areas that do not already have a big investment in an existing coding scheme. This should make it easier to achieve the stated goals of using SNOMED CT to provide NHS staff with consistent and easily understood information about a patient's medical history, illnesses, treatments and test results wherever and whenever it is needed. The terminology can be used for diagnosis, treatment, sharing of information and for research.

The Dictionary of Medicines + Devices (DM+D) provides unique identifiers and associated textual descriptions for medicines and devices. It has been developed for use throughout the NHS (in hospitals, primary care and the community) as a means of uniquely identifying the specific medicines or devices used in the diagnosis or treatment of patients. The dictionary provides a link to SNOMED CT terminology used in clinical systems.

Connecting for Health claim the following benefits for the use of SNOMED CT:

- patients knowing that everyone in the NHS they meet will be using the same language to talk about their condition and treatment
- a single and comprehensive system of terms, centrally maintained and updated for use in all NHS organisations and in research
- greater consistency in communication of patients' clinical records
- simplified data entry and retrieval
- reliable analysis and research based on a common understanding of health terms and concepts stored in a coded form (rather than as free text)
- good links to recognised health classifications (International Classification of Disease and Related Health Problems) and surgical classifications (from the Office of Population, Censuses and Surveys) to assist research into disease and treatment.

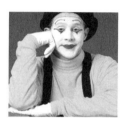

Pause for thought

1 How many people do you share data with?
2 Do you know that everyone codes to the same standards?
3 Or if you are not currently using codes, how will you ensure that you are using the same codes as everyone else?

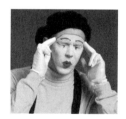

Key points from this chapter

- Standards are boring, but vital.
- Some standards are not your problem.
- Data standards are crucial.
- Everyone needs to use the same standards.
- Primary care has many years' experience with Read Codes.
- The proposed coding and classification scheme for the NHS is SNOMED CT, which is to be used across the whole NHS.

8 Keep information safe

Information governance

Information governance has been defined as

'a framework for handling information in a confidential and secure manner to appropriate ethical and quality standards.'

NHS Scotland, 2004

Information governance is guided by five basic principles on the protection and use of patient information provided by the Department of Health.

- Don't use patient information unless absolutely necessary.
- Use the minimum necessary.
- Access on a strict need-to-know basis.
- Be aware of responsibilities.
- Understand and comply with the law.

This is not specifically an IT issue. However, the increased adoption of IT and clinical staff's occasional unfamiliarity with it can raise particular governance issues. It makes it easier to store and distribute information – for better, for worse.

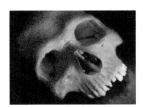

Zombie Warning!

There is a common view that information governance was invented because of computers.

In reality, the use of IT forced the NHS to consider many issues that it should have addressed many years before.

You may like to think of IT as a barium meal for information governance. Increased use of technology may reveal existing challenges in governance.

The problems of information governance outside of computers were highlighted in the Bristol and Alder Hey inquiries. In both cases IT is offered as part of the solution.

Data protection

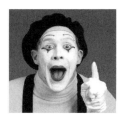

Tip: The 1998 Data Protection Act

The 1998 Act removed the distinction between paper and electronic records for data protection purposes.

The first UK Data Protection Act was established in 1984 to deal with protection of data held on computers. In 1998, this was replaced by a much more comprehensive Act that brought us into line with Europe.

The major differences in the new Act, which became law in 2000, are as follows:

- the Act now covers certain types of manual records (including all health records) as well as electronic records. There are transitional arrangements concerning manual records between now and 2007
- the definition of 'processing' is wider than that in the 1984 Act, and includes the concepts of obtaining, storing and disclosing data. Most actions involving data, including storage, will be included within this definition
- although both the 1984 and 1998 Acts include eight Data Protection Principles, the nature of the principles differs between the two Acts
- the Access to Health Records Act 1990 permitted access to manual health records made after the Act came into force (1 November 1991). The Data Protection Act 1998 permits access to all manual health records whenever made, subject to specified exceptions
- changes to the requirements for notification of processing to the Data Protection Commissioner (formerly the Data Protection Registrar).

Guidance on the 1998 Act, Department of Health, 2000

The law now states that 'anyone processing personal data must comply with the eight enforceable principles of good practice'. It says that data must be:

- fairly and lawfully processed
- processed for limited purposes
- adequate, relevant and not excessive
- accurate
- not kept longer than necessary
- processed in accordance with the data subject's rights
- secure
- not transferred to countries without adequate protection.

The eight principles of data protection, Information Commissioner
(Data Protection Act, 1998)

Personal data cover both facts and opinions about the individual. They also include information regarding the intentions of the data controller towards the individual, although in some limited circumstances exemptions will apply. With processing, the definition is far wider than before.

All processing of data to which the Act applies must comply with the eight principles. The first principle is particularly important as it emphasises that processing must be fair and lawful in the context of the common law and other UK legislation. Generally it will be complied with if all the following conditions are met:

- the common law of confidentiality and any other applicable statutory restrictions on the use of information are complied with
- the data subject was not misled or deceived into giving the data
- the data subject is given basic information about who will process the data and for what purpose
- in the case of health data, one of the conditions in both Schedule 2, which deals with any personal data, and Schedule 3 to the Act, which deals with sensitive personal data, is satisfied.

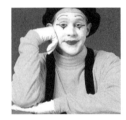

Pause for thought

Are you sure you are operating within the law?

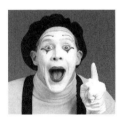

Tip

If not, then seek out your local Caldicott Guardian, whose job it is to protect patient confidentiality, and who should be able to advise you.

Confidentiality

According to the GMC, one of the key responsibilities of a doctor is to respect and protect confidential information (GMC Standards of Practice, 2001).

Other professional groups have similar rules: as a registered nurse or midwife, you must protect confidential information.

You must treat information about patients and clients as confidential and use it only for the purposes for which it was given. As it is impractical to obtain consent every time you need to share information with others, you should ensure that patients and clients understand that some information may be made available to other members of the team involved in the delivery of care. You must guard against breaches of confidentiality by protecting information from improper disclosure at all times.

You should seek patients' and clients' wishes regarding the sharing of information with their family and others. When a patient or client is considered incapable of giving permission, you should consult relevant colleagues.

If you are required to disclose information outside the team that will have personal consequences for patients or clients, you must obtain their consent. If the patient or client withholds consent, or if consent cannot be obtained for whatever reason, disclosures may be made only where:

- they can be justified in the public interest (usually where disclosure is essential to protect the patient or client or someone else from the risk of significant harm)
- they are required by law or by order of a court.

NMC, 2004*

The first issue arising from these codes is: what constitutes confidential information?

Within the NHS, it is defined thus:

A duty of confidence arises when one person discloses information to another (e.g. patient to clinician) in circumstances where it is reasonable to expect that the information will be held in confidence. It:

- is a legal obligation that is derived from case law;
- is a requirement established within professional codes of conduct; and
- must be included within NHS employment contracts as a specific requirement linked to disciplinary procedures.

Department of Health, 2003

Is that helpful? I thought not!

The official guidance makes a distinction between patient-identifiable data and non-identifiable data. This creates its own set of difficulties.

Anonymised data may still be identifiable from other factors. For example, it would be difficult to identify a patient from a diagnosis of asthma, as this is very common. As we refine the diagnosis and combine it with other factors such as age, gender and ethnicity, we may quickly provide a unique profile of a patient, who could be identified.

In practice, the duty of care on a clinician to protect the data is not removed by anonymising it. Some of the anonymised data used routinely for disease

---

* © Nursing and Midwifery Council. Reproduced with permission.

surveillance in public health, including for example sexually transmitted disease data, are among the most sensitive.

Alternatively, if we diagnose a rare condition, that may be unique within a practice or primary care trust.

The Department of Health guidance on confidentiality states that:

> It is extremely important that patients are made aware of information disclosures that must take place in order to provide them with high-quality care. In particular, clinical governance and clinical audits, which are wholly proper components of healthcare provision, might not be obvious to patients and should be drawn to their attention. Similarly, while patients may understand that information needs to be shared between members of care teams and between different organisations involved in healthcare provision, this may not be the case and the efforts made to inform them should reflect the breadth of the required disclosure. This is particularly important where disclosure extends to non-NHS bodies.
>
> Department of Health, 2003

It seems optimistic to me that patients will necessarily see clinical governance and clinical audits as 'wholly proper components of healthcare provision'. The guidance identifies three distinct cases and provides advice on how to deal with each case in the form of decision trees:

1 where it is proposed to disclose confidential information in order to provide healthcare
2 where the purpose isn't healthcare but it is a medical purpose as defined in legislation
3 where the purpose is unrelated to healthcare or another medical purpose.

> Department of Health, 2003

The advice is reproduced in Figures 8.1–3. The grey area in all these cases comes where patients refuse to give consent for disclosure of information. Clinicians may be faced with a choice between doing the best for their patient and their obligations to the broader healthcare system. The official advice seems to me to be plausible but fails to deal with the complexities faced by clinicians in practice:

> Patients generally have the right to object to the use and disclosure of confidential information that identifies them, and need to be made aware of this right. Sometimes, if patients choose to prohibit information being disclosed to other health professionals involved in providing care, it might mean that the care that can be provided is limited and, in extremely rare circumstances, that it is not possible to offer certain treatment options. Patients must be informed if their decisions about disclosure have implications for the provision of care or treatment. Clinicians cannot usually treat patients safely, nor provide continuity of care, without having relevant information about a patient's condition and medical history.
>
> Department of Health, 2003

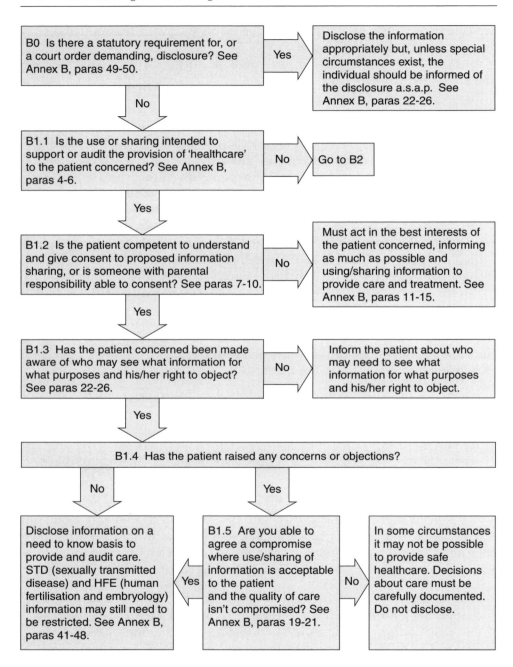

Figure 8.1 Disclosure model: where it is proposed to share confidential information in order to provide healthcare*

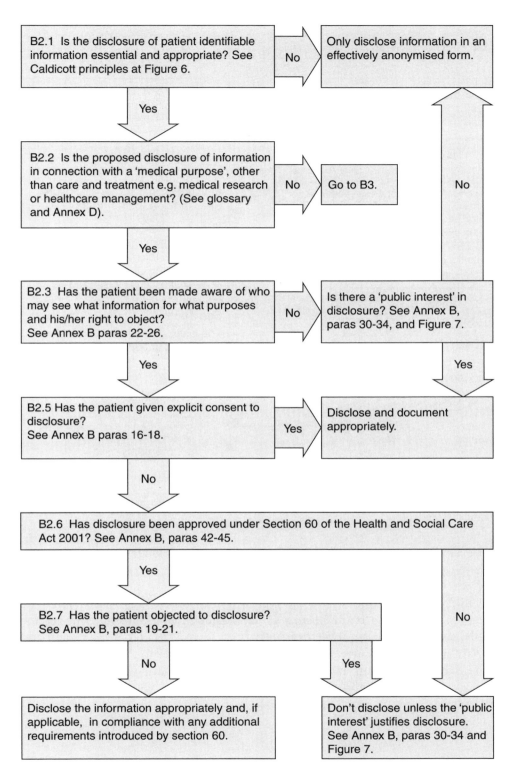

Figure 8.2 Disclosure model: where the purpose isn't healthcare but it is a medical purpose as defined in the legislation*

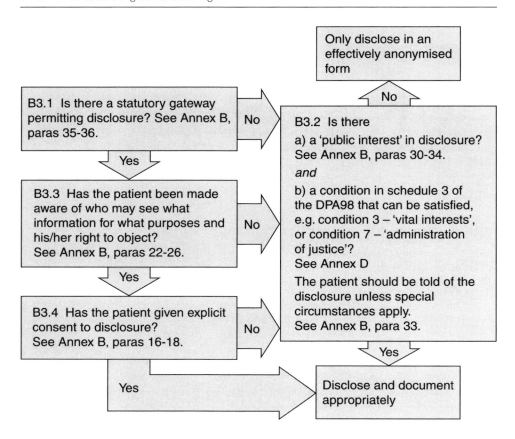

Figure 8.3 Disclosure model: where the purpose is unrelated to healthcare or another medical purpose*

For example, clinicians find themselves all the time with inadequate information, balancing that against the good of the patient, e.g. in drop-in centres, NHS Direct and when called out at night.

Ultimately, the law does state that there are situations where consent cannot be obtained for the use or disclosure of patient-identifiable information, yet the public good of this use outweighs issues of privacy. Section 60 of the Health and Social Care Act 2001 currently provides an interim power to ensure that patient-identifiable information, needed to support a range of important work such as clinical audit, record validation and research, can be used without the consent of patients.

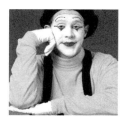

Pause for thought

If 'Clinicians cannot usually treat patients safely, nor provide continuity of care, without having relevant information about a patient's condition and medical history', how safe are all of our health services away from the regular GP surgery?

(*This is taken from the Department's advice on confidentiality.*)

When a patient discloses private information to their doctor, or another individual clinician, they do not necessarily expect that information to be available to another member of their healthcare team.

They may go further and explicitly state that they wish it to remain confidential to that individual clinician. In the modern healthcare system, however, care is often a team activity and may require information sharing among the team. The official advice states:

Patients generally have the right to object to the use and disclosure of confidential information that identifies them, and the need to be made aware of this right. Sometimes if patients choose to prohibit information being disclosed to other health professionals involved in providing care, it might mean that the care that can be offered can be limited and in extremely rare circumstances that it is not possible to offer certain treatment options. Patients must be informed if their decisions about disclosure have implications for the provision of care or treatment.

Department of Health, 2003

The tradition of the relationship between a patient and their registered GP is very strong in the UK. Most patients would be happy to share more personal information with their own GP than with another clinician. Equally, they would be happier to share it with a clinician who is directly involved in their treatment than one who is not, or a manager who is using the information for a purpose that has a less direct impact upon the care of that patient.

In other systems, e.g. Australia, where there is a much weaker link between patients and a specific clinician, the emphasis upon patient privacy is stronger. On a recent visit, I interviewed a GP about his patients, many of whom had serious conditions including HIV/AIDS. He said:

'My patients would come to me for treatment relating to their AIDS or hepatitis. They would visit another GP closer to home for their routine medication, and that physician may not know of their condition.'

This raised serious issues for me around the balance between confidentiality and the risk to the patient's health. Upon return to the UK, I queried this with a UK GP, and asked him if the position was similar here. He replied that:

> 'If a patient is diagnosed with a condition such as AIDS by an outside agency, for example an STD clinic, that diagnosis would not necessarily be reported to their GP.'

Whilst this reflects a vital sensitivity to the need for confidentiality around diseases which may carry a significant stigma in society, it undermines the principle that UK GPs have overall responsibility for the care of their patients, and that this principle is not necessarily carried over to other conditions that may carry equal stigma, e.g. mental health problems.

Gillies, 2003

There is a clear trade-off between disclosure of information to professional colleagues on a 'need-to-know' basis and the desire for patient privacy. However, there is a clear principle that patients' consent must be sought for disclosure, and that that consent must be properly informed.

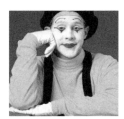

Pause for thought

If you believed that a close relative was suffering from a mental health problem and needed medical help, with whom would you be prepared to share that information?

1 their GP
2 an anonymous clinician
3 an anonymous non-clinical NHS employee
4 the police

Increasingly, patient care is a multi-agency activity, involving several health agencies, social care agencies and, increasingly, voluntary agencies.

There is a tension between providing the best possible information, especially in a multi-agency situation, to facilitate the best possible care and the need to respect confidentiality.

As defined in the Data Protection Act 1998, medical purposes include, but are wider than, healthcare purposes. They include preventive medicine, medical research, financial audit and management of healthcare services. The Health and Social Care Act 2001 explicitly broadened the definition to include social care.

Experience shows that there are different attitudes to information collecting.

In the healthcare sector generally, there is a view that the more information collected the better, since this provides a richer picture of the health of the patient.

Particularly in primary care, a wide range of factors may influence the health of the patient, and the immediate symptoms and stated reason for consulting the doctor may not be the most significant factors.

This has sometimes had a negative influence on GP systems, which have tended to become 'sinks' for information, with little thought as to when the information may be retrieved and in what form.

By contrast, social workers tend to be much more minimalist in their information collection, preferring to emphasise that only relevant and targeted information, which is linked to specific courses of action, is collected. This has been explained in terms of the fear of litigation. This derives from cases where, following a failure of care, it can be shown that information was available and not acted on.

The PCT may find the social care agencies less than grateful for a drip feed of inconclusive pieces of information, relating to problems with children at risk or mental health patients housed in the community.

System usage must therefore be defined within agreed protocols, where it is clearly defined at what point action is required on the part of an individual professional or manager. However, it is recognised that even this may not be enough to *sell* the system if a culture of fear exists.

There are also different attitudes to confidentiality.

Although health data are appropriately regarded as 'sensitive', the information in most child health records is not as sensitive as that relating to children being classified as *at risk*. Much child health data are routine, e.g. recording the occurrence of childhood diseases. These data carry no stigma.

The very act of recording that a child may be at risk is extremely sensitive and changes the nature and context of all information regarding that child. For example, a child arriving at A&E with a fracture, with no history or label attached, is likely to receive only sympathetic treatment. The knowledge that this child has been deemed to be *at risk* changes the nature of the information from a simple clinical diagnosis with consequences limited to treatment of the injury, to potentially crucial evidence of significant abuse.

Thus, professional and parental attitudes to the information are likely to be fundamentally different. There is no significant need for excessive confidentiality over an incident such as a fracture arising from a genuine accident, unless there is a belief that the injury is caused by deliberate harm.

PCTs are increasingly likely to function as teams of practices. Each practice is already operating much more as a team than was the case maybe ten years ago. Thus, increasingly, healthcare is managed as a team activity. In most circumstances, it is professionally acceptable for all members of a team involved in the healthcare of a patient to have access to all relevant information.

However, the number of professionals involved in the process of care for a child deemed to be at risk may be considerable, and the degree of their involvement may vary significantly. Therefore, it is appropriate to define a hierarchical model of access to sensitive information on a *need-to-know* basis. For example, teachers and police officers may be involved in the process, but need to have only partial knowledge. Within a school, there may be further differentiation between teachers designated to deal with child abuse cases, teachers with direct pastoral responsibility, such as form or year tutors, and class teachers.

Department of Health guidance on joint working highlights the following principles:

- information to be shared must be purposeful and justified
- information should be specifically geared to the task it is intended to serve
- the information should be sufficient and sharing should exclude unnecessary material
- information should normally only be shared with the informed consent of the subject
- information should be shared as part of appropriately planned and managed procedures
- information should only be shared within agreed 'information communities'
- personal identifiers should be removed wherever possible
- agencies should take responsibility for ensuring proper procedures for compliance
- standards must be established to ensure that technologies used in information sharing are fully fit for the purpose.

> Draft guidance and regulations on the section 31
> partnership arrangements, Department of Health, 1999

More recent policy has increasingly treated social care as part of healthcare. However, this does not cover other agencies, e.g. voluntary agencies or the police. While the police have no general right of access to health records, there are a number of statutes that require disclosure to them and some that permit disclosure. These have the effect of making disclosure a legitimate function in the circumstances they cover. In the absence of a requirement to disclose there must be either explicit patient consent or a robust public interest justification. What is or isn't in the public interest is ultimately decided by the courts. Where disclosure is justified it should be limited to the minimum necessary to meet the need and patients should be informed of the disclosure unless it would defeat the purpose of the investigation, allow a potential criminal to escape, or put staff or others at risk.

Most NHS organisations will have procedures to deal with such situations, and clinicians should refer to these to protect themselves and their patients.

Freedom of information

The Freedom of Information Act only applies to public authorities, including NHS trusts, and companies that are wholly owned by public authorities.

Public authorities are obliged to provide information:

- through a 'publication scheme'
- in response to requests made under the general right of access.

A publication scheme is both a public commitment to make certain information available and a guide to how that information can be obtained. All publication schemes have to be approved by the Information Commissioner and should be reviewed by authorities periodically to ensure they are accurate and up to date.

When responding to requests, there are set procedures that public authorities need to follow. These procedures include:

- the time public authorities are allowed for responding to requests. In general, organisations have 20 working days to respond to requests
- the fees or amount that public authorities can charge for dealing with requests. Public authorities are not obliged to deal with requests if the cost of finding the information exceeds a set amount known as the appropriate limit
- public authorities need not comply with vexatious or repeated requests.

The Act also recognises that there are valid reasons for withholding information by setting out a number of exemptions from the right to know.

It is worth remembering that the Freedom of Information Act does not require organisations to reveal personal data in breach of the Data Protection Act and if an individual clinician receives a request under the Freedom of Information Act, they should refer it to their Caldicott Guardian or Information Governance Lead.

What are the risks?

Once we accept that as clinicians we have a professional duty to protect patient information, it becomes a duty to assess and manage risks arising from the way that we process and store those data.

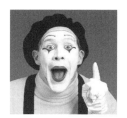

Tip: Risk associated with IT

In general, storing information using IT exposes it to greater risk.

HOWEVER, the technology also provides much better facilities for managing and reducing that risk.

Because you have these facilities available to you, you have a legal and ethical duty to use them. Not to do so could be considered professionally negligent, if you do not take the steps that your peer group of professionals would normally take.

Electronic data face a different range of risks from paper-based data. In general, they are less at risk from accidental loss, damage or wear and tear. The technology itself can also help to protect the patients' information if used correctly. On the other hand, there are new and different threats to electronic data.

You should consider how to protect your patients' information against:

- accidental damage
- unauthorised access
- and malicious damage.

Some necessary actions will not be your job, but many risks can be reduced by good habits.

Protecting your patients' information against accidental damage

Paper-based records have always been at risk of accidental damage through the threats of fire and flood. Additional risks include loss due to incorrect filing. Each of these risks has a corresponding risk for computerised records. Computers can be destroyed by fire or flood or even, *in extremis*, cups of coffee! Similarly, records may be filed under a wrong name or deleted accidentally. It is much easier accidentally to delete a computerised record than accidentally to throw away a physical record.

Computers have additional risks, due to their need for an external power supply, and their technological complexity. Clinical coding makes incorrect data entry potentially more likely, as different clinicians may wish to use different codes for the same condition.

However, the most significant difference is that the technology can provide a means of managing the risks.

As we have a duty to keep patient information secure, so there is a duty to make the best use of technology to protect the information from accidental damage. The following table shows how we can protect against the identified risks:

Table 8.1 Protecting information against identified risks

Risk	*Management*
Flood	Regular backups Remote storage of backups
Fire	Regular backups Remote storage of backups
Power failure	Continuous power supply Regular backups
Equipment failure	Regular backups
Incorrect data entry	Data validation Data entry protocols
Accidental deletion of files	Confirmation dialog boxes

A good backup strategy is essential. A typical strategy might look like Table 8.2.

Table 8.2 A typical backup strategy

Day	Task
Monday	Incremental backup
Tuesday	Full backup
Wednesday	Incremental backup
Thursday	Incremental backup
Friday	Full backup removed to remote secure destination
Saturday	Incremental backup
Sunday	Incremental backup

Using this schedule gives you daily protection against equipment failure or a power supply failure that beats your power supply backup, or against accidental deletion. It means that you are never more than a week away from full data in the event of a major catastrophe.

Procedures to make backup copies of the patient record system must be:

- appropriately planned to ensure that a valid recent copy can be recovered
- regularly, correctly and consistently carried out
- verified by checking the integrity of the backed-up data (on every occasion).

Used backup disks and tapes should be replaced with new media at regular intervals, taking account of the manufacturer's recommendations on the antici-pated working life of the media used. Old backup media should be re-formatted or physically disrupted so as to render any data on them unrecoverable. If the backup procedure offers a choice of backing up different parts of the system, the routine backup procedure should always include a backup of the audit trail.

The organisation should have a policy on data entry to minimise risks in this area. The policy may allow another person to make entries in the patient records on behalf of the responsible healthcare professional. The information on which such entries are based may be a written note, a dictated message or a verbal report by the healthcare professional responsible for the observations or interventions recorded.

Entries made in this way must be:

- transcribed to the computerised record by an authorised trained person who ascribes the entries to the healthcare professional who wrote or dictated the notes
- monitored in accordance with the practice policy on data entry to ensure the accuracy and correct attribution of the entries made.

The clinical system should record details of who, what and when, in an audit trail.

Audit trails should be capable of detecting tampering and should be secured against deletion. If reports and correspondence are received electronically from outside the practice, the practice policy should include procedures to ensure that:

- all information received is seen by the person responsible for the original request or by another doctor acting on his or her behalf
- the information received is filed in the computerised record of the patient to whom it relates.

Finally, confirmatory dialog boxes are an essential part of any system design. They seek to stop you accidentally doing something with unforeseen consequences.

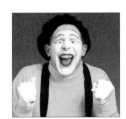

Smile !

I prefer to think of them as 'Have you lost your presence of mind?' boxes.

It's usually worth taking a deep breath before telling the computer that 'No, of course, I haven't!' and telling it to 'Get on with what I asked you to do' by clicking on 'Yes'.

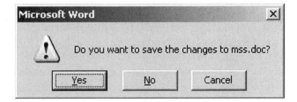

Figure 8.4 A 'Have you lost your presence of mind?' dialog box

Protecting your patients' information against unauthorised access

Electronic records are at risk not just from people who want to read them, but people who thinks it's fun to see if they can.

Paper-based records have always been at risk of unauthorised access. In order to obtain access, however, the interloper has had to be in the presence of the records.

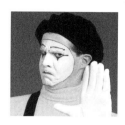

Warning!

Now with the advent of computer networks, people seeking unauthorised access can do so remotely. What is more, some people do it just for fun.

The first line of defence against unauthorised access is password protection. The Department of Health code of conduct offers the following advice

For all types of records, staff working in offices where records may be seen must:

- Shut/lock doors and cabinets as required.
- Wear building passes/ID if issued.
- Query the status of strangers.
- Know who to tell if anything suspicious or worrying is noted.
- Not tell unauthorised personnel how the security systems operate.
- Not breach security themselves.

Manual records must be:

- Formally booked out from their normal filing system.
- Tracked if transferred, with a note made or sent to the filing location of the transfer.
- Returned to the filing location as soon as possible after use.
- Stored securely within the clinic or office, arranged so that the record can be found easily if needed urgently.
- Stored closed when not in use so that contents are not seen accidentally.
- Inaccessible to members of the public and not left even for short periods where they might be looked at by unauthorised persons.
- Held in secure storage with clear labelling. Protective 'wrappers' indicating sensitivity – though not indicating the reason for sensitivity – and permitted access, and the availability of secure means of destruction, e.g. shredding, are essential.

With electronic records, staff must:

- Always log out of any computer system or application when work on it is finished.
- Not leave a terminal unattended and logged in.
- Not share logins with other people. If other staff have need to access records, then appropriate access should be organised for them – this must not be by using others' access identities.
- Not reveal passwords to others.
- Change passwords at regular intervals to prevent anyone else using them.

- Avoid using short passwords, or using names or words that are known to be associated with them (e.g. children's or pet names or birthdays).
- Always clear the screen of a previous patient's information before seeing another.
- Use a password-protected screensaver to prevent casual viewing of patient information by others.

Department of Health, 2003*

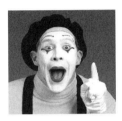

Tip

Passwords should be longer than six characters and use a mixture of letters and numbers to make them as difficult to guess as possible. A truly random combination of five letters offers more than 10^{169} combinations, and including numbers increases this to 10^{186} combinations. This is increased further if you mix case. However, as we find it difficult to remember a random sequence, we tend to use our pet dog's name or similar!

The other good practice is to change passwords regularly – and always if you suspect that it may be *at risk.*

Protecting your patients' information against malicious damage

Paper-based records have always been at risk of malicious damage. Fire and flood may be initiated deliberately.

Computers are attractive objects in themselves, both to thieves and also to people who write viruses to attack computers. In Salford, Greater Manchester, in the mid-1990s, one practice was so worried about theft from premises that their entire computer system had to fit onto one laptop that could be removed at night.

Generally, however, while physical security is certainly an issue, the threat from viruses is a greater risk. In recent years, the NHSNet has been attacked and breached by the 'I love you' virus, and the Blaster worm.

The following advice is given to general practices:

- Disks received from outside the practice should be checked for viruses by effective and regularly updated anti-virus programmes;
- Files received from outside the practice by electronic transfer should also be checked for viruses.

BMA GPC/RGCP, 2000

---

* © Crown copyright. Reproduced under licence with permission.

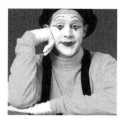

Pause for thought

In the late 1980s, at the height of public ignorance and fear over AIDS, when the current epidemic in sexually transmitted infections was just beginning, my boss sent round a memo about 'data hygiene'.

However, if you don't mind the rather messy image of data as bodily fluids, vital but dangerous if infected, there are some helpful analogies.

- With whom do you share data?
- Do you know who they share their data with?
- If you share data with people, then you are exposed to all the same risks that they are.

It's worth thinking about these issues in relation to your own situation.

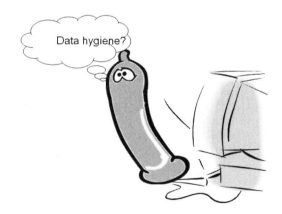

Figure 8.5 Data hygiene: safe sex for computers?

Every NHS organisation should have a security policy that takes full account of the need for confidentiality as well as authentication and integrity of the computerised patient record system. The security policy should take account of local circumstances and risks, but should specifically address the points under the headings below.

- Security policy
- Security organisation
- Asset classification and control
- Personnel security

- Physical and environmental security
- Communications and operations management
- Access control
- System development and maintenance
- Business continuity management
- Compliance

The policy should recognise the need for data entry to be restricted to properly trained and authorised people. It must take full account of the need for entries to be accurate, complete and attributed to the person responsible for the observations or interventions recorded. When considering the issue of authentication, all staff should be aware that they may be held liable for the content and accuracy of information that appears to have been entered by them or on their behalf. It is therefore important that the security features of the system and procedures followed by the practice combine to minimise the risk of a record entry being accidentally or fraudulently attributed to the wrong user.

It may be necessary to prove that an entry was or was not made by the person to whom it is attributed. This means that, since most record entries are logged as being the responsibility of the individual whose password is currently entered, it should never be acceptable for an entry to be made into a record when someone else has logged into the system. More generally, it is essential that all users:

- have a unique user identity and password
- keep their password secret and do not divulge it to other users for any reason
- change their passwords at frequent intervals
- log out of workstations when their task at that workstation is finished and never leave a workstation logged in, but unattended.

The policy should ensure that the organisation has a clearly laid-out disaster recovery plan. This will need to address the temporary replacement of the organisation's electronic functions with paper-based alternatives, the retention and subsequent entry of these temporary records into the electronic record system when it becomes available again, and the extraction of essential information from ancillary systems such as any electronic appointment book's backup.

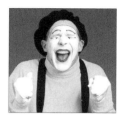

Smile !

The NHS is working towards BS7799 as an information security standard.

I refuse to call this a tip because I can't possibly imagine what use it could be to you.

If you go to the kind of parties where you can drop this into conversation, then the tip you need is that you are going to the wrong kind of parties!

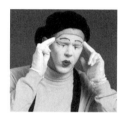

Key points from this chapter

This chapter is all derived from the five basic principles.

- Don't use patient information unless absolutely necessary.
- Use the minimum necessary.
- Access on a strict need-to-know basis.
- Be aware of responsibilities.
- Understand and comply with the law.

9 Involve the patients in decision making

Consent

In recent years, the view of consent has changed significantly, as greater emphasis has been placed upon respecting patients' autonomy. Much of this has happened in response to two particular scandals that have received massive publicity in the UK.

- Between 1988 and 1995, two heart surgeons at Bristol Royal Infirmary carried out 53 operations – and over half of the young patients died (Kennedy 2001).
- The scandal at Alder Hey emerged almost accidentally when heart specialist Professor Robert Anderson revealed at the Bristol inquiry that a store of children's hearts was kept at Alder Hey (Redfern 2001).

There was also an alarmingly similar case in Canada, where 12 infants and children died during or after cardiac surgery between February and December of 1994 at the VCHC, Winnipeg (Manitoba Health 2001).

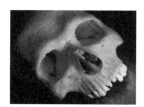

Zombie Warning!

When I was in hospital, I heard a doctor say he had come to 'obtain' my consent.

The view that informed consent is 'obtained' from patients and that the signature is all the evidence required flies in the face of current legislation, policy and evidence from patients.

Like all good zombies, in spite of this, it persists.

A common theme in the subsequent enquiries was that informed consent was not adequately obtained in these situations. Traditional views of consent as a signature on a form have been challenged as a result.

The Department of Health has produced guidance on what constitutes informed consent following the reports into Bristol and Alder Hey. That advice states that:

> For consent to be valid, it must be given voluntarily by an appropriately informed person (the patient or where relevant someone with parental

responsibility for a patient under the age of 18) who has the capacity to consent to the intervention in question. Acquiescence where the person does not know what the intervention entails is not 'consent'.

To give valid consent the patient needs to understand in broad terms the nature and purpose of the procedure. Any misrepresentation of these elements will invalidate consent. Where relevant, information about anaesthesia should be given as well as information about the procedure itself.

Clear information is particularly important when students or trainees carry out procedures to further their own education. Where the procedure will further the patient's care – for example taking a blood sample for testing – then, assuming the student is appropriately trained in the procedure, the fact that it is carried out by a student does not alter the nature and purpose of the procedure. It is therefore not a legal requirement to tell the patient that the clinician is a student, although it would always be good practice to do so. In contrast, where a student proposes to conduct a physical examination which is not part of the patient's care, then it is essential to explain that the purpose of the examination is to further the student's training and to seek consent for that to take place.

Although informing patients of the nature and purpose of procedures enables valid consent to be given as far as any claim of battery is concerned, this is not sufficient to fulfil the legal duty of care to the patient. Failure to provide other relevant information may render the professional liable to an action for negligence if a patient subsequently suffers harm as a result of the treatment received.

Department of Health guidance on informed consent
(Department of Health, 2001)

The requirements of the legal duty to inform patients have been significantly developed in case law during the last decade. In 1985, the House of Lords decided in the Sidaway case that the legal standard to be used when deciding whether adequate information had been given to a patient should be the same as that used when judging whether a doctor had been negligent in their treatment or care of a patient: a doctor would not be considered negligent if their practice conformed to that of a responsible body of medical opinion held by practitioners skilled in the field in question (known as the 'Bolam test'). Whether the duty of care had been satisfied was therefore primarily a matter of medical opinion. However, Sidaway also stated that it was open to the courts to decide that information about a particular risk was so obviously necessary that it would be negligent not to provide it, even if a 'responsible body' of medical opinion would not have done so.

Since Sidaway, judgements in a number of negligence cases (relating both to the provision of information and to the standard of treatment given) have shown that courts are willing to be critical of a 'responsible body' of medical opinion. It is now clear that the courts will be the final arbiter of what constitutes responsible practice, although the standards set by the health professions for their members will still be influential.

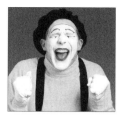

Smile !

When I was in hospital I started talking to the doctor who had come 'to obtain my consent'.

He was very concerned to do the right thing, but pointed out that the advice to provide information on all the risks was not always easy to implement. For example, if you have a nervous patient about to go down to theatre, is the last thing they want to hear before they set off that the anaesthetic might kill them?

Bad joke answer: Yes, the last thing they want to hear before they go down to theatre is *that the anaesthetic might kill them.*

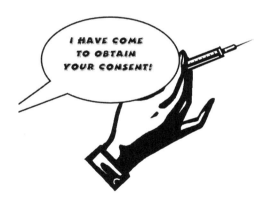

Figure 9.1 Obtaining consent . . .

In considering what information to provide, you should try to ensure that the patient is able to make a balanced judgement on whether to give or withhold consent. Case law on this issue is evolving. It is therefore advisable to inform the patient of any 'material' or 'significant' risks in the proposed treatment, any alternatives to it, and the risks incurred by doing nothing. A recent Court of Appeal judgement stated that it will normally be the responsibility of the doctor to inform a patient of 'a significant risk which would affect the judgement of a reasonable patient'.

The General Medical Council has gone further, stating in guidance that doctors should do their best to find out about patients' individual needs and priorities when providing information about treatment options. The guidance also emphasises that if the patient asks specific questions about the procedure and associated risks, these should be answered truthfully.

> In the very rare event that the health professional believes that to follow the guidance in the previous paragraphs in full would have a deleterious effect on the patient's health, the GMC guidance states that this view, and the reasons for it, should be recorded in the patient's notes. When such concerns arise it is advisable to discuss the issue within the team caring for the patient. In an individual case the courts may accept such a justification but would examine it with great care. The mere fact that the patient might become upset by hearing the information, or might refuse treatment, is not sufficient to act as a justification.
>
> Some patients may wish to know very little about the treatment which is being proposed. If information is offered and declined, it is good practice to record this fact in the notes. However, it is possible that patients' wishes may change over time, and it is important to provide opportunities for them to express this. The GMC guidance encourages doctors to explain to patients the importance of knowing the options open to them, and states that basic information should always be provided.
>
> General Medical Council guidance to doctors (GMC, 2004)

Following the report of the Manitoba Paediatric Cardiac Surgery Inquest, the following advice was provided:

> Consent can be either expressed or implied; it can be verbal or written; it can be qualified or unqualified; and, of course, it can be refused. Having the patient sign the consent form is a familiar and important ritual of medical practice, but the form is simply evidence in written form that the patient confirms that he/she understand the explanations that have been given and agrees with the proposed course of action.
>
> A number of legal principles have come to underpin the concept of informed consent. It is their interpretation and application in complicated factual and sensitive ethical situations where the potential for controversy arises. The five criteria for informed consent identified by Canadian courts are:

- consent must be genuine and voluntary;
- the procedure must be a legal procedure;
- the consent must authorize the particular treatment or care as well as the particular care giver;
- the consenting patient must be competent to consent, i.e. must be legally of age and have the mental capacity to give consent; and
- the consent must be informed.

On the last criterion, information must be provided in language that the patient can understand. The obligation to provide the information rests with the physician who is to carry out the treatment. The information that must be provided includes: the nature of the proposed treatment, anticipated effects, material or significant risks, alternatives available and any information regarding delegation of care. Nurses regularly witness the signing of consent forms, but in doing so they are not testifying to the adequacy of the explanation which the physician gave to the patient.

Manitoba Health, 2001

While this guidance is helpful, it tends to focus upon what informed consent is not, perhaps reflecting the impact of litigation in this area.

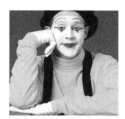

Pause for thought

What do you think constitutes informed consent, and what do you do to make sure that the patient has provided it?

Accessibility to information for patients

We have already seen that IT can help us provide information for patients to allow them make informed choices. However, many patients are from groups who may have problems in accessing information; for example, older patients may have poor vision and find written material difficult to read. The Campaign for Plain English has highlighted that much information is provided in language that is overly complex.

For example, consider the following extract chosen randomly from the CHD NSF.

Standards One and Two: Reducing heart disease in the population*

Standards

The standards for prevention of CHD are that:

Standard one

The NHS and partner agencies should develop, implement and monitor policies that reduce the prevalence of coronary risk factors in the population, and reduce inequalities in risks of developing heart disease.

Standard two

The NHS and partner agencies should contribute to a reduction in the prevalence of smoking in the local population.

---

* © Crown copyright. Reproduced under licence with permission.

Interventions

The interventions that should be put in hand to improve the cardiac health of the local population are:

Effective policies

development and implementation of a comprehensive local programme of effective policies for reducing smoking, promoting healthy eating and physical activity, and for reducing overweight and obesity – led by the NHS in collaboration with partner agencies

Health & Health Inequality Impact Assessments

public agencies are encouraged to estimate and report publicly on the likely impact of their major decisions on the cardiac health of the local population, including inequalities

Smoking

development of effective local smoking cessation services by the NHS (see HSC 1999/087)

Community development

local organisations should facilitate and co-ordinate the establishment of community development programmes that address at least one of the determinants of coronary heart disease in the most disadvantaged, hard-to-reach and high-risk communities that they serve.

Exemplary employers

Public agencies are encouraged to provide healthy workplaces by:

* developing organisational policies which help promote job control
* making a variety of healthy foods readily available to staff
* providing staff with opportunities for physical activity
* ensuring that their premises have no-smoking policies
* encouraging staff and visitors to use alternatives to the car.

Service models

The service models for delivering effective prevention policies and programmes should include:

The Health Improvement Programme:

Local players, co-ordinated by the HA, should work together to produce a Health Improvement Programme (HImP) that:

* makes clear the priority they attach to improving health and to reducing inequalities in health
* refers explicitly to the recommendations in the Director of Public Health's annual report
* refers explicitly to the Local Equity Profile

- specifies the actions for which each organisation takes responsibility and is held accountable for delivering
- creates local links to relevant prevailing national policies
- specifies the structure, process and outcome measures by which local delivery of the policies will be judged.

Key stakeholders

Local players will establish a local implementation team to develop and oversee the implementation of the local delivery plan to put this NSF into practice. The team should consult and involve key stakeholders.

Health Impact Assessment

Local players are encouraged to undertake and make public a prospective health impact assessment of major policy decisions that are likely to have a direct or indirect effect on cardiac health. Retrospective assessments or evaluations of policy will help to monitor how a policy is affecting or has affected health following its implementation and to modify or inform future direction.

Local Equity Profile

Directors of Public Health are expected to produce an Equity Profile for the population they serve. The Equity Profile is intended to identify inequalities in heart health and in access to preventive and treatment services. It will comment on the needs of individuals and groups, particularly those for whom special consideration is warranted. It will complement HIAs, and will directly inform the HImP.

Smoking cessation

HAs, with PCGs/PCTs, will be expected to establish specialist smoking cessation services for smokers who wish to quit. The services should aim to target disadvantaged communities, young people and pregnant women and should be available in a variety of settings. Services should be high profile, accessible and accept self-referral or referral by primary and secondary healthcare professionals and dentists, pharmacists, *NHS Direct,* schools and voluntary organisations. The services will feature support, advice and follow-up to individuals or groups and will offer one week's free nicotine replacement therapy (NRT) to smokers least able to afford it. Members of the primary healthcare team will be expected to provide advice to smokers opportunistically.

Community development

A community development approach helps communities to make their own decisions about how to achieve better health for themselves, their families and the wider community. Professionals are required to act as facilitators, rather than imposing an agenda on the community.

HAs, LAs and PCGs/PCTs need to work together, so that there is at least one community development project with a focus on CHD under way in one of the most deprived communities in every local authority area. Health visitors will be a vital resource in securing successful community development.

Workplace policies
The NHS and LAs should develop and implement policies to protect and improve the health (including the heart health) of staff, and to report progress regularly to their Boards and Councils.

Immediate priorities
The immediate priorities for implementing this area of the NSF are:

• by April 2001, Health Authorities will introduce specialist smoking cessation clinics, helping 150,000 people
• delivering the early milestones.

Milestones
The milestones marking progress in implementing this area of the CHD NSF for reducing the risk of heart disease in the population are:

Milestone 1
By October 2000 all NHS bodies, working closely with LAs, will:

• actively participate in the development of the HImP
• have agreed their responsibilities for and contributions to specific projects identified in the HImP
• have a mechanism for being held to account for the actions they have agreed to deliver as part of the HImP
• have a mechanism for ensuring that progress on health promotion policies is reported to and reviewed by the Board
• have identified a link person to be a point of contact for partner agencies.

Milestone 2
By April 2001 all NHS bodies, working closely with LAs, will:

• have agreed and be contributing to the delivery of the local programme of effective policies on: a) reducing smoking; b) promoting healthy eating; c) increasing physical activity; and d) reducing overweight and obesity
• have a mechanism for ensuring all new policies and all existing policies subject to review can be screened for health impacts
• as an employer, have implemented a policy on smoking
• be able to refer clients/service users to specialist smoking cessation services, including clinics
• have produced an equity profile and set local equity targets.

This extract scores 30 on the Flesch reading ease score that rates text on a 100-point scale; the higher the score, the easier it is to understand the document. For most standard documents, a score of approximately 60 to 70 is deemed to be an acceptable score.

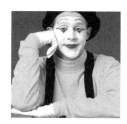

Pause for thought

Do you know whether information you produce for patients is readable and comprehensive?

Readability scores only tell part of the story. Technical terms, abbreviations and acronyms can all make text inaccessible to patients.

For older patients, simply reading the words can be a challenge. According to the RNIB: 'There are two million people with sight problems in the UK. Good design can make your websites, information materials, . . . accessible to them'. This is no longer just good practice, it is the law under the Disability Discrimination Act. Websites present a particular challenge: the next time the corporate IT department insists that any information that you place on the web must conform to NHS guidelines, they *may* be doing you a favour!

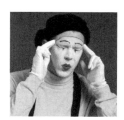

Key points from this chapter

- Patient consent has become even more important since the events at Bristol and Alder Hey.
- IT and the Internet in particular provide a range of resources that can help inform patients, but
- Any information provided for patients needs to be accessible to all.

10 Conclusions

We have seen that the NHS is about to embrace IT in a systematic way for the first time. This book has tried to give you a realistic impression of what is in store. It has shown where the benefits can be achieved and where there are implications that will require NHS staff to work in different ways in order to achieve the benefits.

Ten years ago, I went to a GP practice to help a group of GPs who were not keen to embrace the new technology. I walked in and they immediately started to tell me their woes:

'It's not working for us. It's more effort than it's worth,' they said.
'I know,' I replied.
'No, no, you're not listening to us: it's not working!' they said.
'No, you're not listening, I know it's not working for you,' I replied.
'No, no, listen . . . what did you say?'
'I know it's not working for you. What's more, even if you do all the things I suggest over the next year, it still won't work for you, but if you do all the things I suggest over the following year, you might see some benefits, and if you carry on after that, you will reach a point where you might even think it's worth all the effort!'
'But I thought you were supposed to come and sell the idea of using the stuff to us?'
'I think I just did!'

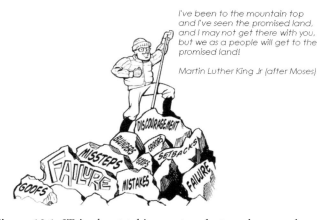

I've been to the mountain top and I've seen the promised land, and I may not get there with you, but we as a people will get to the promised land!

Martin Luther King Jr (after Moses)

Figure 10.1 IT is about taking us to a better place . . . honestly!

I think this is a microcosm of the NHS in 2005: we're in for a rough couple of years, but if we persist we may get to a better place, and wonder how we ever managed without it (or even IT!), just like I currently do every time I pay a bill from my desk in my study or, even better, book a flight to somewhere exotic.

References

Blom Cooper L, Hally H and Murphy E (1995) *The Falling Shadow: one patient's mental healthcare* (1979–1993). HMSO. London.

BMA GPC/RCGP (2000) *Good Practice Guidelines for General Practice Electronic Patient Records*, The Joint Computing Group of the General Practitioners' Committee and the Royal College of General Practitioners. BMA, London.

Celler BG *et al*. Using information technology to improve the management of chronic disease. *Medical Journal of Australia*. **179**: 242–6.

Data Protection Act (1998) Chapter 29. Part 1 of Schedule 1. HMSO, London.

Department of Health (1990) *The Care Programme Approach for People with a Mental Illness*. HMSO, London.

Department of Health (1997) *The New NHS: modern dependable*. HMSO, London.

Department of Health (1998) *Information for Health: a national information strategy for local implementation*. HMSO, London.

Department of Health (1999) *Draft Evidence and Regulations on the Section 31 Partnership Arrangements (for consultation from September to October 15, 1999) Part 1*. HMSO, London.

Department of Health (1999) *National Service Framework for Mental Health: modern standards and service models*. HMSO, London.

Department of Health (2000) *Data Protection Act 1998. Protection and Use of Patient Information*. HMSO, London.

Department of Health (2001) *Mental Health Information Strategy*. HMSO, London

Department of Health (2002) *Delivering 21st Century IT Support for the NHS*. Information Policy Unit. HMSO, London

Department of Health (2003) *Confidentiality: NHS Code of Practice*. HMSO, London

Department of Health NHS Executive (1992) *Information Management and Technology Strategy* HMSO, London.

Freedom of Information Act (2000) Chapter 36. HMSO, London.

General Medical Council (2001) *Good Medical Practice*. GMC, London.

General Medical Council (2004) *Confidentiality: Protecting and Providing Information*. GMC, London.

Gillies AC (2003) *What Makes a Good Healthcare System?* Radcliffe Medical Press, Abingdon.

Glover G (1999) How much English Health Authorities are allocated for mental health care. *British Journal of Psychiatry*. **175**: 402–6.

Kennedy I (2001) *The Report of the Public Inquiry into Children's Heart Surgery at the Bristol Royal Infirmary 1984–1995: learning from Bristol*. HMSO, London.

Manitoba Health (2001) *The Report on the Manitoba Paediatric Cardiac Surgery Inquest*. Review and Implementation Committee, Manitoba Health, May 2001.

NHS Scotland (2004) Information Governance. Available on-line at http://www.isdscotland.org/ (accessed December 2005).

Nursing and Midwifery Council (2004a) *The NMC Code of Professional Conduct: Standards for Conduct, Performance and Ethics*. NMC, London.

Nursing and Midwifery Council (2004b) *Guidance on Record Keeping*. NMC, London.

Peto J, Gilham C, Fletcher O and Matthews F (2004) The cervical cancer epidemic that screening has presented in the UK. *The Lancet*. **364**: 249–56.

Protti D (2005) *A World View*, available online at www.npfit.nhs.uk (accessed February 2005).

Redfern M (2001) *The Report of The Royal Liverpool Children's Inquiry*. HMSO, London.

Standing Nursing and Midwifery Advisory Colmmittee (SNMAC) (1999) *Addressing Acute Concerns*. Mental Health Nursing, London.

Wanless D (2002) *Securing Our Future Health: taking a long-term view*. Final Report, HM Treasury, London.

Wing JK, Curtis R and Beevor A (1996) *Health of the Nation Outcome Scales*. Report of development. Royal College of Psychiatrists Research Unit, London.

Bibliography

Access to Health Records Act. HMSO, London.

Benner P (1984) From novice to expert: excellence and power in clinical nursing practice. Addison Wesley, California.

Deming WE (1986) *Out of the Crisis.* MIT Press, Boston.

Department of Health (1988) *Access to Medical Records.* HMSO, London.

Department of Health (1989) *Caring for People.* HMSO, London.

Department of Health (1989) *Working for Patients.* HMSO, London.

Department of Health (1990) *Community Care in the Next Decade and Beyond.* HMSO, London.

Department of Health (1991) *The Patient Charter.* HMSO, London.

Department of Health (1992) *The Health of the Nation.* HMSO, London.

Department of Health (1995) *Building Bridges: arrangements for inter-agency working for the care and protection of the mentally ill.* HMSO, London.

Department of Health (1995) *OPCS Survey of Psychiatric Morbidity in Great Britain.* Report. HMSO, London.

Department of Health (1995) *Proposed Criteria for SMI.* HMSO, London.

Department of Health (1995) *The Report into Clinical Standards Advisory Group on Schizophrenia.* HMSO, London.

Department of Health (1998) *A First Class Service: Quality in the new NHS.* HMSO, London.

Department of Health (1998) *Our Healthier Nation: a contract for health.* HMSO, London.

Department of Health (1998) *Modernising Mental Health Services: safe, sound and supportive.* HMSO, London.

Department of Health (1998) *Modernising Social Services: promoting independence, improving protection, raising standards.* HMSO, London.

Department of Health (1998) *Partnership in Action: new opportunities for joint working between health and social services.* HMSO, London.

Department of Health (1998) *Working Together: securing a quality workforce for the NHS.* HMSO, London

Department of Health (1999) *Making a Difference.* HMSO, London.

Department of Health (1999) *The Caldicott Report.* HSC1999/012. HMSO, London.

Department of Health (2001) *Consent – What You Have a Right to Expect: a guide for children and young people.* HMSO, London

Department of Health (2001) *Essence of Care.* HMSO, London.

Department of Health (2001) *Good Practice in Consent Implementation Guide: consent to examination or treatment.* HMSO, London

Department of Health (2001) *Guidance on Consent.* HMSO, London

Department of Health (2001) *Good Practice in Consent: achieving the NHS Plan commitment to patient-centred consent practice.* HSC 2001/023. HMSO, London

DHSS (1986) *A National Strategic Framework for Information Management in the Hospital and Community Health Service.* HMSO, London.

Disability Discrimination Act (1995) Chapter 50. HMSO, London.

Gillies AC (1995) The computerisation of general practice: an IT perspective. *Journal of Information Technology.* 10(1): 75–85.

Gillies AC (1996) Improving patient care in the UK: clinical audit in the Oxford Region, *International Journal for Quality Assurance in Health Care.* 8(2): 141–52.

Gillies AC (1997) *Improving the Quality of Patient Care.* John Wiley, Chichester.

Gillies AC (1997) The year 2000 problem in general practice: an information management based analysis, *Journal of Health Informatics.* **3**(3 and 4): 147–53.

Gillies AC (1998) Computers and the NHS: an analysis of their contribution to the past, present and future delivery of the National Health Service. *Journal of Information Technology.* **13**(8): 213–29.

Gillies AC (1998) *Information and IT for Primary Care.* Radcliffe Medical Press, Abingdon.

Gillies AC (2000) Assessing and improving the quality of information for health evaluation and promotion. *Methods of Information in Medicine.* **39**(3): 208–12.

Gillies AC (2000) Information support for general practice in the new NHS. *Health Libraries Review.* **17**(2): 91–6.

Gillies AC (2001) *Excel for Clinical Governance.* Radcliffe Medical Press, Abingdon.

Gillies AC (2001) *Presenting Health with PowerPoint.* Radcliffe Medical Press, Abingdon.

Gillies AC (2001) Risk management issues associated with the introduction of EHRs in primary care. Published at www.primarycareonline.co.uk. Now unavailable; copies on request from the author.

Gillies AC (2002) *Health Care Databases: how to use and build them.* Radcliffe Medical Press, Abingdon.

Gillies AC (2002) *Providing Information for Health for Primary Care.* Radcliffe Medical Press, Abingdon.

Gillies AC (2002) *Using Research in Nursing.* Radcliffe Medical Press, Abingdon

Gillies AC (2002) *Using Research in Primary Care.* Radcliffe Medical Press, Abingdon.

Gillies AC (2003) *What Makes a Good Healthcare System?* Radcliffe Medical Press, Abingdon.

Gillies AC and Howard J (2003) Managing change in process and people: combining a maturity model with a competency-based approach. *TQM & Business Excellence.* **14**(7): 797–805.

Gillies AC and Rawlings GR (1998) Can computers improve the Health of the Nation?' *Journal of Health Informatics.* **4**(2): 147–53.

Gillies AC, Ellis, B and Lowe N (2001) *Building an Electronic Disease Register.* Radcliffe Medical Press, Abingdon.

Goddard J, Alty A and Gillies AC (2001) A case study in mental health informatics: barriers to integrated care pathways. *IT in Nursing.* **13**(3): 12–15.

Healthcare Commission (2004) NHS Performance Ratings 2003/2004, available online at www.healthcarecommission.org.uk (accessed June 2005).

Race Relations (Amendment) Act (2000). HMSO, London.

Romanow RJ (2002) Commission on the Future of Health Care in Canada. *Building on Values: the future of health care in Canada.* Health Canada, Ottawa.

Shaw NT and Gillies AC (2001) *Going Paperless.* Radcliffe Medical Press, Abingdon.

Storey L, Howard J and Gillies AC (2002) *Competency in Healthcare.* Radcliffe Medical Press, Abingdon.

Index